10668659

ON THE FAR SIDE
Of The Curve

A STAGE IV COLON CANCER SURVIVOR'S JOURNEY

**Marshall Co Public Library
@ Benton
1003 Poplar Street
Benton, KY 42025**

WAYNE COOKE

Baker + Taylor

SEP 0 1 2010

Copyright © 2009 Wayne Cooke
All rights reserved.

ISBN: 1-4392-5240-8
ISBN-13: 9781439252406
Library of Congress Control Number: 2009907743

Visit www.booksurge.com to order additional copies.

Dedicated to my parents, Gilbert and Lottie Cooke, my wife Pat, my son Scott, his wife Cristina, their two children Xavier and Rafael, my daughter Kelly, my siblings, Dean, Janet, Al, Dan and Jim, and all of the family members, doctors and friends who have supported and strengthened me throughout this journey.

Foreword

I first met Wayne Cooke in January 2004 when he came into my office with his wife, Pat, for a consultation for a recent diagnosis of colon cancer that had spread to his liver. He proceeded to follow my guidance and we have now worked together for over five and a half years. I would consider his case a classic example of how to treat stage IV colon cancer.

His positive attitude in his fight against cancer is an inspiration for many cancer patients. Mr. Cooke shows how one can treat cancer as a chronic disease and to live with cancer while maintaining a good quality of life, including singing in his church choir, European choir tours, holidays with family and many memorable overseas trips.

He teaches us that while cancer has many side effects, in spite of cancer, one can still live a life of wisdom, faith, and love. Also having a supportive wife, Pat, and family makes it much easier to live with cancer.

This book ought to be read by everyone who has cancer or has a loved one with cancer. I hope that reading this book helps many patients and their families to get the healing lessons that they need so that everyone gets on the far side of the curve as Mr. Cooke has done.

Peter I. Yi, MD, FACP
Medical Oncologist, Princeton Medical Group, University Medical Center at Princeton
Clinical Assistant Professor of Medicine at Robert Wood Johnson Medical School

Prologue

I am a stage IV colon cancer survivor, so far. After having been diagnosed with colon cancer that had metastasized to my liver almost
six years ago and having undergone three major surgical procedures
and over seventy cycles of various chemotherapy and infusional treatments, I am now considered stable. Some people are starting to call
me "the Miracle Man." Several oncologists have recently used terms
such as "one of a kind," "unique," and "on the far side of the curve" to
describe my survivorship. But after all of my treatments and surgeries, I am still left with four non-operable pulmonary nodules in my
left and right lungs. So my doctors are telling me that I should start
to consider my cancer a chronic disease- to be treated and lived with,
but not cured.

Along this journey I have had a number of experiences and learned
a number of lessons that I feel might be useful to others who are facing cancer or other life-threatening diseases. I have had to rethink my
life and am probably a better person now than I was six years ago.
And I have had the support of a lot of people: my wife, my son and
daughter, my siblings, a lot of friends and some very good doctors.

I have had to face up to a number of questions including: How
does one deal with the uncertainty of living with cancer? Why me?
Or on the other side of that coin, maybe not Why me? But why not
me? Why can't I be the one to survive? But how have I been able to
survive a supposedly terminal disease and live this long while others

have not? Hopefully, I can try to answer these and other pertinent questions in this journal.

In that regard, I have also taken a look at what I may have learned from growing up in small town Ohio, the second of six children, or my time at the University of Michigan, the US Navy or thirty years at IBM. This past history on some of the events in my life and my reactions along the way may shed some light on my ability to cope with this disease.

I have also included a timeline of the medical events and treatments that I have gone through. And I have included, at the end of the story, a summary of a number of what I feel are the most important lessons I have learned.

And perhaps my experiences can give others hope for the future.

So let's get started.

Timeline

2000
Aug Normal colonoscopy

2003
Nov Diagnosed with Stage IV colon cancer
Dec Colon resection at University Medical Center at Princeton

2004
Feb-Sept Chemotherapy with Princeton Medical Group
Oct Liver resection at Memorial Sloan Kettering Cancer Center (MSKCC), NYC
Dec Resume chemotherapy at Princeton Medical Group

2005
Feb In remission

2006
Jan Recurrence in liver
Mar Right liver resection at MSKCC, NYC
May In remission
July Pulmonary nodule growth in Left and Right lungs
Aug Resume chemotherapy at Princeton Medical Group
Nov Pulmonary nodules stable

2007

Feb   Start "chemo holiday"

Aug   Growth in pulmonary nodules in Left and Right lungs

Aug   Resume chemotherapy at Princeton Medical Group

2008

Feb   Start another "chemo holiday"

Aug   Growth in pulmonary nodules, resume chemotherapy

2009

Feb   Reduced chemotherapy: maintenance treatments with Avastin

CHAPTER 1:
I've Got Cancer!

"AT LEAST YOU WON'T NEED A BAG"

It all started in the fall of 2003 on the Tuesday before Thanksgiving. I had volunteered to help out at the Trenton Soup Kitchen that day with other members of the Princeton United Methodist Church. Afterwards, I was feeling good about myself as I went to an appointment with a local surgeon, Dr. Thomas Davidson, to check out some rectal bleeding problems that I was having.

I didn't expect to find anything too serious as I had been in general good health, beside the somewhat usual high blood pressure and high cholesterol stuff, and had had a normal colonoscopy from Dr. Davidson three years prior, in August 2000. I had been to see my GP sometime earlier and he found nothing that would cause my symptoms and said that if they persisted I should go to see Dr. Davidson. So here I was. I thought at worst he would find a hemorrhoid or something like that. He had fit me in with the last appointment of the day.

At first he checked me out and didn't seem to find anything serious. Then he said "look, you're here and I'm here and I've got some time, so let's do a more comprehensive test." He gave me a fleet enema, sent me to the bathroom to get ready, and when I came back he performed a sigmoidoscopy, which is a test that looks at the lower third of the colon.

Much to my surprise, he said that he found something that he did not like and was going to take a biopsy. I asked what that meant, and he said that there was a possibility of cancer, but he knew about the clean colonoscopy just three years prior and that cancer polyps were not supposed to form that quickly. Nonetheless, he said that he was going to send the sample out and that with Thanksgiving coming up we would not get the results back until Friday. My wife, Pat, and I know him personally (we both had kids who had gone to college together), and he said that he would call us at home Friday evening.

As I was leaving his office, his nurse said, "Well, at least you won't need a bag," referring to the bag that many people end up with after having had a colostomy or rectal surgery. At the time, I thought it was a cruel joke, but I realize now that she was trying to make a tense situation more positive. They had indicated that the growth that they found was far enough up the colon that a straightforward colon resection was possible, and a more comprehensive colon-rectal job would not be required. She was trying to make me feel good about a possible bad situation.

That night, when I told Pat about my visit to Dr. Davidson, she was surprised. She was unaware of my symptoms and also unaware that I had gone to see him that day. And neither of us was aware that it would be the start of a process that she would be involved with almost every day of my life for the next six years. We were both suddenly very apprehensive about our future together.

THE BAD NEWS

Thanksgiving that year was at my Brother Jim's house in center city Philadelphia. Thanksgiving had always been a big holiday in the Cooke family, starting from my early days growing up in Bowling Green, Ohio. I was the son of a college professor with four brothers and a sister. Jim is my youngest brother and his family and mine frequently alternate Thanksgiving between my home in Princeton, New Jersey and his.

This year was his turn and my wife and I were there along with my son, Scott and his wife Cristina. My brother, Jim, his wife, Janet, and one of his two daughters, were there as well. Our daughter, Kelly, was not, since she was living in London at the time with her husband. We had been having a very nice time and then at the end of the evening, I shared with them the news that I was expecting the results of a test the next day, and that we would keep them advised. A pleasant day ended on a somber note.

Friday was a very long day. Pat and I anxiously awaited the phone call from Dr. Davidson. That evening the call came, and it was not the news that we wanted to hear. I did indeed have colon cancer. We were devastated to say the least. While he does not normally have office hours on the weekend, Dr. Davidson said that he would like to see us in his office the following morning.

That Saturday morning, Pat and I had a long discussion with him about colon cancer, the first of many discussions we would have with doctors over the next six years. Dr. Davidson wanted to schedule some more tests to determine the extent of my disease, including a colonoscopy and a series of CT Scans, and also to discuss the surgery that he was recommending: a colon resection to take out about 18 cm of the colon, including the diseased section. We left that session down-hearted, not knowing just how to proceed with our lives. Pat may not have known it yet, but she was already settling in to the role of Caregiver. *(See Lesson 1)*

That Sunday we had the first of many discussions with one of the ministers at our church. At the time we were not prepared to talk openly to many people about my condition but wanted him to know what was going on. It felt comforting to have a minister aware of my situation. At this time we were almost afraid to talk to anyone else.

The next week the dates for the surgery and the follow-up tests were scheduled, including a colonoscopy, CT scans and pre-admission testing. When they attempted to do the colonoscopy they could not safely get by the area with the tumor so they reverted to a barium enema as a fall-back: it was probably the worst test that I endured over this whole process because of the discomfort involved. Although many people do not like the colonoscopy, I heartily recommend it over the barium enema.

My wife and I were leading pretty busy lives at that point in time. We were busy as realtors for the Coldwell Banker office in Princeton where my wife was one of the top agents, and we had two closings and a number of other real estate- related activities coming up in the next two weeks. We typically divide up the work with Pat taking care of the customer contacts, interface to the real estate community, and taking customers out in the car. I take care of transaction management and the MLS related stuff. This division of activities worked out pretty well over the years that we have worked together and was especially relevant the various times that I lost my hair because of chemo since I could do a lot of the computer work at home and people did not have to know how I looked.

I also sing in the Princeton United Methodist Church choir and with Voices Chorale, a mixed chorale group in the area, and had a full agenda of Christmas concerts coming up. So we started to plan how we would get through the time until I completed my surgery and recovery. At that time, I didn't expect to be out long.

The first of the Voices Chorale concerts was scheduled the next weekend and I decided to sing in it. It was an outreach concert in the community hall of the nearby town of Yardley, Pa. At the time, I was the bass section leader, responsible for the care and feeding of the baritone/bass section (also for taking attendance, keeping track of people's scheduled absences, scheduling sectional rehearsals as necessary, etc). I had a short discussion with another one of the basses, Al

Chan, regarding my condition and asked him if he would temporarily mind taking over my duties until I returned.

At the time I expected to be out of commission with the surgery for two or three months at most. I also told him that due to the schedule of my surgery, I would not be able to sing the next three concerts that were on the docket for December. I enjoyed being able to sing in the Yardley concert, not knowing that I would not only miss the remaining December concerts, but many others over the next few years. And little did Al know that he was agreeing to be bass section leader not just for the next few months, but in actuality for the next five years.

The next weekend, my wife and I went to a local holiday party, where I ran into a doctor who was a cancer specialist at the Cancer Institute of NJ located in New Brunswick. I briefly discussed my situation with him, and he said that if the cancer was contained in the colon it was a straightforward operation and follow-up, and that the chances of survival were good. If it had advanced beyond that stage, then it could be a long haul and survival was more uncertain.

My colon surgery was scheduled for the following Thursday.

CHAPTER 2:
And It's Stage IV!

MORE BAD NEWS

The Monday before my surgery, Dr. Davidson called to say that the results of the CT scans were back and they were not good. They showed that there were three spots on my liver: two small spots on the right side and a larger one on the left. This meant that the cancer had moved from the colon, through the colon wall, into the blood stream and metastasized in the liver. This is called Stage IV colon cancer and is about as bad as it gets. Colon cancer has been categorized in stages ranging from Stage 0, the earliest stage to Stage IV, the most advanced. Unfortunately, by the time I was diagnosed, I was already at the most advanced stage.

Dr. Davidson said that while he had done liver resections for cancer over his 35 plus years of surgery, he did not specialize in hepatic (liver) surgery, and we might want to look for a liver specialist if my situation resulted in having cancer surgery on the liver. We also needed to consider whether we should schedule both colon and liver surgeries at the same time as this could be potentially convenient but was a more involved and dangerous surgical procedure.

This raised a lot of questions. What were we to do now? Colon surgery as scheduled later in the week or something else? We were neophytes to this situation. We were dealing with a lot of new terms, did not have a plan and were pretty confused. That evening

I contacted the cancer doctor that I had seen the prior weekend and asked if he had any advice. He said that he would try to line me up with a liver surgeon at his center in New Brunswick, and would send out an email that night.

On Tuesday we were advised that we could see the liver specialist in New Brunswick the next morning, which was the day before my scheduled colon surgery on Thursday. This was indeed a positive break, because normally they scheduled new patients out weeks in advance. I called Dr. Davidson's office to tell him about this appointment, particularly because I was supposed to start the bowel prep for my surgery on Wednesday morning. They told me that if I started the prep at noon after the morning appointment, it would be ok. So Wednesday morning Pat & I went off (with my scan films under my arm) to the Cancer Institute of New Jersey in New Brunswick.

The liver specialist recommended that I take a step-by-step approach. He said that having surgery on three tumors on both sides of the liver at the same time was more difficult and with more risk involved than with fewer tumors, and that the new chemotherapy treatments just coming available might be able to shrink or eliminate one or more of the spots. He would recommend having the colon surgery first, and then have chemo to attack the liver spots and keep the liver surgery open as a future option. We thought that was a good, solid approach, and left his office knowing that, at least, we had a plan for the immediate future. *(See Lesson 3)* We called Dr. Davidson's office and told them that we were good to go for surgery the next day, and I went home to start the bowel prep procedure.

COLON SURGERY-DECEMBER 2003

I believe that one has anxious moments anytime one has a major surgery. I had had two previous major operations at the Medical Center at Princeton where the colon surgery was being done: one in 1977 for a tumor in my left parotid, which resulted in the whole left side of my face being cut open, (and turned out to be benign), and the second in 1983 for a ruptured appendix, which was originally misdiagnosed as a heart attack (but that is a whole different story). So I was familiar with the hospital. The anesthesiologist, Mary Beth, was a member of our church and it was comforting to see her in the surgical suite. And although I am told the surgery went on for some while, it was successful.

My wife, Pat, my daughter, Kelly, (who had flown home from London), and my son, Scott, who lives about an hour away with his wife in Westfield, but works locally at Bristol-Myers Squibb, were all there when I recovered. Dr. Davidson had taken out 18 centimeters of the lower colon and appeared to get all of the local cancer. My immediate recovery went fine. I was tired but feeling pretty good.

A couple of days later, however, my body had a reaction. My pulse rate jumped and they could not seem to get it back to normal. I was moved from the oncology floor to the telemetry unit where they have the ability to continuously monitor your vital signs. They could not find a normal room for me so I was put in a small space at the end of the hall in front of a private room near the red light for an exit door.

Then began two of the most difficult days of all of my hospital stays. The high heart rate caused anxiety and I could not get comfortable at all. Being on the telemetry floor, I had a monitor pack on my chest to go along with pulsating boots, an oxygen feed, IV drip, catheter, etc. I was a mess. And to top it off, they would come in to check my vital signs every few hours, so I could not get any sleep. They sent me down to the radiology floor for a number of new scans and tests to see if anything from the surgery had caused the elevated heart rate, and didn't find anything. They tried additional procedures throughout the night, all of which failed to alleviate the problem.

That night I remember looking up at the red exit sign on the door the whole time. Since people had to go through my temporary space to get to the patient in the next area, his wife and the nurses kept going by my bed all night to care for him. I was miserable. I remember the next morning calling Pat at about 7:30. "Get me out of here!" I told the nurse that I was leaving. She was a bright spot in the whole thing. First, she told me that if I left without being formally discharged, my insurance would not cover the bills, so she did not recommend escape as a course of action. But, most of all, she told me that the person in the space behind me was being moved out and that I would be moved into that space later in the day. Hurrah. My wife later told me that getting that "crisis" call from me at 7:30 in the morning was one of the toughest things that she has had to deal with during this whole process.

After I was moved to the new room, things started to look up. An interventional cardiologist, Dr. James Beattie, came to see me and told me that, if I agreed, there was a procedure that he could try that might bring my pulse rate down. The procedure would be administered locally, but they would be monitoring it from the control room on the telemetry floor. After he left the friendly nurse told me that she had worked with patients that had had the procedure, that she would be with the doctor the whole time, and that I would be ok. I agreed to proceed. And you know what? The procedure went well, my pulse rate came down to about 60 and it has remained there ever since. I had been stretched to the limit, but was beginning to have some hope.

CHAPTER 3:
Stretched to the Limit

There are times in your life when you feel that you are stretched to the limit. When your adrenalin gets really pumped up and you really feel stressed out. I am sure that there are many jobs where this happens regularly, such as firemen, police, first responders, or top gun pilots, but most of us probably don't have that many times when it happens to us.

Looking back on my total cancer experience, this two day hospital stay in the telemetry ward was probably the worst part. I was trying to think back to other such experiences that might have helped me prepare for such an event and could only think of a few in my lifetime. Nothing popped up in my early days in Bowling Green, Ohio, my high school days, or even University of Michigan. All of that seemed to be the normal stuff of growing up. But later in life some stressful situations started to come to mind, some of which were of my own making and are worth commenting on.

1956: THE SUPPLY OFFICER'S MISTAKE

I believe the first time I had such an experience was in 1956 when I was a Supply Officer in the USN serving on the USS Leary DDR 879. I had joined the ship in Beirut, Lebanon and after returning to the States for a while, we set out for a Caribbean exercise. One of my responsibilities was paying the crew twice a month and I had to keep a safe supplied with the amount of money I might need for the cruise. I was used to keeping large sums of money since I had previously been the Disbursing Officer on the USS Albany CA 123, a heavy cruiser and frequently had over $500,000 in cash in my custody. I would balance the safe periodically, normally keeping the daily cash separate from the bulk cash reserve. So after the first payday at sea, I tried to balance my cash. I was $10,000 short.

I tried several other ways to balance the cash and always ended up with the same result. I was mortified, picturing court martial, and all of the other things they had told us at Supply Corps School happened to dishonest supply officers. What was I to do? I was a well regarded Supply Officer and had finished as one of the top students at the Supply Corps School in Athens, Georgia the previous summer. I remember sitting for a while thinking about what I could do.

Then I looked up and saw the money bag that I kept stored out of the way on an upper shelf in the supply office. It was the bag that I used when I picked up cash at the local bank at the Norfolk, Virginia Naval Base, where we were stationed. It was in an unsecured location, and anyone who worked in the supply office or walked by could access it. I knew that I could not trust leaving money around the supply office, since I had previously had a small amount stolen from the drawer of my desk, for which I was personally responsible to pay back. So I quickly jumped up from my chair, and pulled down the money bag, and lo and behold, there was a package of twenty dollar bills totaling $10,000. I had left it there by mistake the last time that I picked up cash at the bank.

I was exalted to say the least, and my Navy career was "saved." I don't remember then or now how I ever left the money in the bag at the time, but I remember the flow of adrenalin that came with that experience. I never told anyone in the Navy about this event and went on to complete a successful three year career.

NOVEMBER 1973: THE MOUSETRAP BY AGATHA CHRISTIE

In November of 1973, Pat and I were performing in an Agatha Christie play, "The Mousetrap," in a dinner theater production at a local church in Pittsburgh where we had moved to from Detroit in 1969. Dinner was served followed by the first act of the play, then dessert and coffee followed by the second act. We had the parts of Giles and Molly Ralston, the owners of the Monkswell Manor Guest House in England. It is an excellent play and one of the longest running plays in London. We had held the early rehearsals for the play in our basement since our daughter, Kelly, was coming up on a year old and we would not have to get a baby sitter.

Pat & I had met in January 1967 at the ski resort in Boyne Mountain, Michigan and were married at the Shrine of the Little Flower in Royal Oak, Michigan in June 1968.

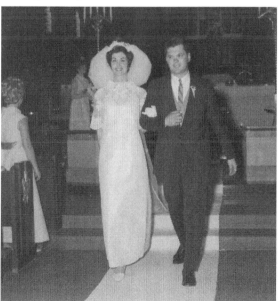

Our Wedding, June 1968

Pat had been a drama major in college and was teaching drama in a Detroit area high school at the time of our marriage, and I had done a lot of musicals in Jackson, Michigan before our marriage. I was working there for IBM at the time as the computer salesman for the Consumers Power Company account, a large public utility in outstate Michigan. The roles of El Gallo in the Fantasticks, the Pirate King in Gilbert & Sullivan's, "The Pirates of Penzance" and Pooh Bah in "The Mikado" were three of my favorites. Pat and I had also performed together in "Guys and Dolls" at the Village Players in Birmingham, Michigan before moving to Pittsburgh. So we both enjoyed doing theater.

During the run of "The Mousetrap," I was promoted by IBM from Marketing Manager of the Mellon Bank account in Pittsburgh to Industry Manager in the Finance Industry Marketing group in Princeton. The Industry Director, my new boss, had already scheduled a fall planning session for his direct reporting managers at the Pocono Manor Hotel in the Poconos and I was expected to attend. The job was one that I had been eager to get and I did not want the play to impact my performance on the new job.

I had it worked out that I could get from the Pocono hotel to the local airport to catch an early-afternoon puddle-jumper and get to Pittsburgh in plenty of time for the Friday evening performance. Then it snowed. I got to the local airport late. The plane was late. Everything was late. And the snow was still coming down. And I was getting worried. The play was due to start at 8PM and I was scripted to be onstage for the first scene. I had to get there in time.

Finally the small plane took off and we made it to the Pittsburgh airport. As I hurried out into the parking lot, I don't remember what time it was but I knew that I was already going to be late for the cast call. Then it hit me. The parking lot was a sea of snow covered mounds. There was 3-5 inches of snow on top of every car. I had a general idea of where I had parked, but for the life of me, I could not find my car. I was totally distraught. I finally started running down the rows of the cars rubbing snow off to hopefully find my car underneath. No luck.

This was before the days of cell phones, so in order to call the church I would have to go back into the airport to find a pay phone and lose a lot of valuable search time. Or I could go back to get a cab to the church. That appeared to be my best option when at long last I found the car under a big pile of snow, got it started and hit the road.

I reached the church just minutes before 8PM. Everyone was relieved, especially Pat who had no idea why I was so late. Fortunately all of my costumes were stored at the church. I sat for a few minutes to recover my senses, gather myself and let my adrenalin settle down, and then the play went on. Several years later while living in Europe, we took our children to see the "original" version of the Mousetrap in London. We felt that, except for their perfect British accents, our version of the play was equal to theirs.

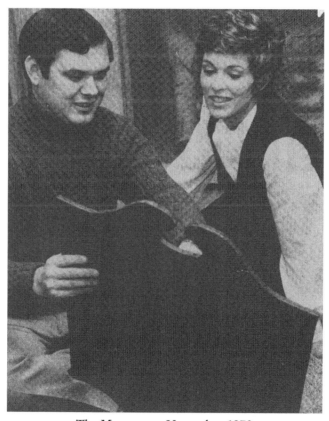

The Mousetrap- November 1973

JUNE 1977: FACE TO FACE WITH A KLM JET

One last such stressful adrenalin generating experience worth commenting about came in 1977 just after we had just moved to Europe for an assignment with IBM in the Netherlands. I was in Paris to make a presentation to the second in command of IBM Europe on a product launch for which I was the responsible manager. He had a reputation for being very tough on new managers. And this was first time I would be meeting him face to face. So I was nervous to start with to say the least.

The presentation went well with few to-dos but took longer than I had planned. I hurried out of the office on Rue St Honore to get a taxi to Charles DeGaulle airport for my 9:00 PM flight to Schipol, the last flight of the day to the Netherlands. I was eager to get back since the container shipment with our household goods had arrived from the States and was due to be delivered to our new home in Holland the following morning. Well, rather than doing the sensible thing of having the office order me a cab, I didn't want to wait for that and instead went out to hail one down in the street. It was a busy rush hour in Paris and there were no available cabs. I raced here and there to try to find a cab stand or an available cab. Time was passing and it was past 8:00. I was running out of time.

Finally I got a cab and in my broken French told the driver to get to Charles De Gaulle airport "Tout-de-suite," very fast. We drove as fast as we could while I thought through the options if I did not make it back on that plane. I could get a hotel room and spend the night and take the first plane out in the morning, I could rent a car and drive five hours to the Netherlands. My mind was racing. We pulled up to the airport at about 10 minutes to 9. I raced through the airport, sped through customs (only a few security checks at this point in time) and arrived at the gate at just 9 PM. The gate was closed, the ramp had been pulled back and the plane doors were shut.

I told the attendant that I had to get on the plane. She politely said that she was sorry but that I was too late. My pulse was racing at top speed. I ran past the surprised attendant, down the stairs and onto the tarmac. The pilot was just ready to start the engines when I ran to the front of the plane and waved my flip chart tube at him. He looked down at me more amazed than anything else. And thank god, it was KLM and not Air France. Then the exterior steps were lowered down and I rushed up and onto the plane. The surprised stewardess did not know quite what to say when I entered and said, "Is this plane going to Amsterdam?" Several of the seated passengers just looked up with amazement and possible amusement. And I knew that I was going to get home in time.

Just thinking about this experience with today's security concerns, I was lucky that I did not end up in jail or something similar. It took the whole of the short flight for my body to calm down. And I made it back in time for the shipment. Of all the things that I have done over my life, this experience of facing down a KLM jet with my attaché case and a flip chart holder has got to rank high on the list.

There are some other experiences that I can think of, but the point is that we, as human beings, are able to sustain periods or events that cause extreme stress and we can make it through. We learn from past experiences how much we can tolerate in new experiences going forward.

What you also learn is that you build your life a day at a time. What you do one day builds on the days before. You can't jump through life. You take each day and make it the best that you can and deal with whatever circumstances that day presents. That way, you can look back from where you are and look on a life filled with many exciting and, hopefully, not too many overly stressful experiences.

CHAPTER 4:
Recovering from Surgery

DECEMBER 2003

After my experience in the telemetry ward, I was moved back to the regular oncology floor and now had a new objective. Christmas was just days away and I wanted to get home by then. So I started questioning my doctor and the nurses about what I had to do to get released. There were the standard things to do. First, I had to be able to get myself up and out of bed. Then I had to be able to get to the bathroom by myself, to suck up a ball in a breathing device, to be able to walk by myself around the nurse's station, and to get back to eating whole food.

I also asked Pat to bring my "hug-me" pillow to the hospital. When you have surgery that cuts the stomach muscles, recovery takes a while. Particularly when you cough or laugh your stomach really hurts. During my ruptured appendix saga in 1983, one of the kind nurses had made what she called a hug-me pillow, which was a blanket of sorts, wrapped up with tape that I could hug against my stomach whenever I coughed or laughed to help moderate the pain. So I knew that I would need the pillow again.

At the time that I had the appendix surgery I was still working as an industry manager for IBM and I clearly remember one day when my boss and a few of my colleagues came to the hospital to see me. We went into a visiting room and they proceeded to tell jokes.

Without my hug-me pillow, with every laugh I would have been in really bad shape.

The net of all this is that I proceeded to follow all of the instructions, to do all of the things that I needed to do and was indeed released from the hospital, with my now normal pulse rate, on the afternoon of December 24th in time for Christmas Eve at home. It was good to be home.

––––––––––

Obviously, I was not up and around much for the remainder of the year, but made it a point to attend church as soon as I could in the New Year. I had been put on the church prayer chain and wanted to thank some of the people who I knew had been praying for me. One cannot overestimate the power of prayer in dealing with serious illnesses. *(See Lesson 4)*

I also made it a point to start learning as much as I could about my disease and its treatments. The Internet is a good source of information, although you have to make sure that what you are reading is up to date, particularly in the case of cancer treatments, which can tend to change quite quickly with the development of new drugs. This was very much the case with metastatic colon cancer.

I had looked over the prior year's annual report on cancer from the American Cancer Society and learned that the five year survival rate for Stage IV colon cancer was less than 10%. This was not a good sign, but was kind of substantiated in a hallway discussion that Pat had had with a doctor in the hospital who indicated that we should get our affairs in order. (She did not share this information with me until some time later, when my outlook had improved.)

But I rationalized this data with the thought that when the five year data was compiled from 1997-2002, it could not include the data from the impact of new chemo drugs, one of which I soon would be taking. I also believed that if 90% didn't make it, that meant that 10% did, and there was no reason for me not to believe that I could be among the ones that did. Regardless, we knew that we were in for a long haul. *(See Lesson 10)*

CHAPTER 5:
My Doctors

DR. YI, I PRESUME: JAN 2004

We now had to find not just a good, but an excellent oncologist to guide us through the next phase of my treatment. And my wife found just such a doctor in Dr. Peter Yi, who had his practice with several other oncologists just minutes from our house. We had our first meeting with him the middle of January 2004. He recommended starting with another comprehensive round of tests: PET scan, CT scan, bone scan, ultrasound, etc., you name it, to try to confirm the extent of my cancer. To schedule all of these tests would take a couple of weeks, following which I was to have a port installed in my upper arm and I would start my first round of chemotherapy.

The chemo program he was recommending was called FOLFOX 4, an abbreviation for 5FU, Leucovorin, and Oxaliplatin. 5FU and Leucovorin had been the standard for colon cancer treatment for many years, but Oxaliplatin was a new drug from France that had been going through trials for several years and had just been approved by the FDA that month. It was so new that he was not yet authorized to administer it in his infusion room. I would have to go to the University Medical Center at Princeton chemo room for treatment until he received his approval. He recommended that we have some follow-up scans after the first three months of chemo to see how I was doing, and, if I could tolerate it, I would continue on the FOLFOX 4 regime for six months.

He also recommended that I make an appointment with Dr. Yuman Fong, a liver surgeon, at the Memorial Sloan Kettering Cancer Center in New York City, just in case we needed to consider liver surgery. He said that he and Dr. Fong had gone through med school together and that "he was the best." I wrote the information down in my book, but did not take any immediate action on that suggestion. Pat and I both felt very comfortable with Dr. Yi.

I have since asked Dr. Yi about the American Cancer Society statistics. He said that he does not normally discuss odds with his patients since he does not want to discourage anyone and it all boils down to how the individual responds to the specific treatment. He did say that he thought that with the current chemotherapy and treatments available, he would think that the odds were more like 25% than 10%. But I would say that by any indicator you would choose to use, for now, I have beaten the odds.

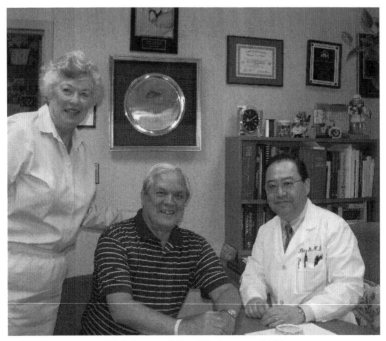

With Pat and Dr. Yi, August 2009

CONFUSING ADVICE

Pat & I were starting to get a lot of free advice. It seems that everyone that we knew had some thoughts on what would be the best treatment; alternative medicines, different surgeons, different hospitals, different chemos that they had heard about. It seemed to be never ending. And we did not want to offend anyone, because at that point in time we did not know yet what the best thing to do was. We were starting to develop a plan, but we were not there yet. It was Pat who came up with the idea that helped us get through this confusing situation.

Dr. Jay Chandler is the surgeon who had done my first two major surgeries in 1977 and 1983. He had retired from his surgical practice but was still consulting and teaching at the hospital in New Brunswick, and was known and well respected in the Princeton community. Pat suggested that we call him for his advice. He not only offered to give us his advice but volunteered to come to our house, since I had not yet had my staples removed from the surgery in December and was not too mobile.

He came over to the house and spent about an hour with us going through various aspects of colon cancer. He had already viewed all of the scans that I had had to date, including some that I had not even received any reports on. He concurred with the advice we had been given by the liver surgeon in December, and knew and approved of Dr. Yi as our oncologist. While he said that I was in for a long haul, he gave Pat & me a good feeling about the program going forward. He did mention that there were some troublesome spots showing up in my lungs that should be checked out. He also offered to be on hand for advice going forward, and we took him up on that offer on numerous occasions over the next five years.

The good news now was that when we received offers of advice from others that did not conform to the program that we were on, we could say that we had consulted with Dr. Chandler on our treatment program and they would back away. We told both Dr. Yi and

Dr. Davidson about this meeting and they both knew Dr. Chandler and approved of the idea. Dr. Yi said that his profession was called a "practice" for a reason and that he did not object to our obtaining any guidance we could get. We were starting to develop a plan. *(See Lessons 2 & 3)*

At church the next Sunday, I saw the doctor from the Cancer Institute of New Jersey and told him what was going on. He suggested that we meet with a colon cancer oncologist there, named Dr. Beth Poplin, to get a second opinion on the chemo plan. She was a specialist in colon cancer and what she could also add to our knowledge was information on any clinical trials that might be underway that it would be helpful to know about. He made the contacts to set up our appointment the following Wednesday morning.

We had that meeting and found Dr. Poplin to be a very knowledgeable and helpful person. She concurred with Dr. Yi's recommendation for the chemo plan. She described in more detail the **FOLFOX** 4 program and how it fit into the overall colon cancer treatments and talked about some of the side effects that they were experiencing with early trials with Oxaliplatin. She described the then- current clinical trials and did not think that any of them would be appropriate for me at that time. We found her very easy to talk to and made it a point to get her opinion several times during the course of my treatment.

CHAPTER 6:
Why Me? Why Did This Happen To Me?

Somewhere along the path, all cancer patients probably ask themselves, "Why did this happen to me?" I know that I did. What you learn is that cancer affects all of us. Of the millions of cells that the body generates every day, a certain number are cancer cells. And in most cases, the body's immune system is able to destroy them. When your immune system breaks down for any reason, then the cancer cells have the chance to take root and multiply, eventually causing problems.

I had shingles in early 2002 along the right side of my waist that caused a rash, pain, some serious swelling and, I am sure, impacted my immune system. I was given some medicine that stopped the rash, but the swelling and pain remained for about six months. It still aches a bit when it rains. I have asked my doctors if there could be any connection with the shingles and my cancer, and have been told that there is no conclusive evidence to indicate that there is. But, I have always wondered whether the shingles attack on my immune system could have paved the way for the cancer.

However, I eventually realized that focusing on the past was not going to help me. What I had to do was focus on what I had now and what I was going to do about it. Getting cancer was not my fault. *(See Lesson 5)* I did have a choice, however, about how I was going to deal with it. I could be passive and let it take its course and control me, or I could be proactive and try to control it. I chose the latter. *(See Lesson 11)*

FREAKED OUT BY THE PET SCAN

I was starting to have a lot of appointments with a lot of different doctors in different locations and found it helpful to keep a notebook of all of my doctor visits. I have maintained that notebook throughout this whole process and have a record of every doctor visit, every test, and every recommendation that we received throughout the past six years. I found it very useful to be able to go back to check out who said what when.

I should not pass by this point in the story without making a comment about the problems that I had with my first PET scan. It is a full body scan that will light up any cancer tumors in your body that are large enough to be detected. You start with about an hour of a dye infusion and then proceed to the machine, which is kind of like an MRI machine, with, I believe, a longer and smaller opening. In my case, the whole test was to take 42 minutes, either 6 minutes at each of 7 positions or 7 minutes at each of 6 positions, I don't remember which. But it was 42 minutes long and the nurse said that she was not supposed to stop the test once it started.

At the time of my first test there, they wrapped me up with my arms at my sides, kind of like a mummy and I was not allowed to move, even if I wanted to. As I started the test, moving into the machine feet first, I could look up at the top of the machine and could see the countdown of the time left at each position. About half-way through I was starting to freak out. I was getting quite claustrophobic and uneasy. Finally at 35 minutes, I had had enough and called for the nurse to come into the room. I was told doing so could compromise the balance of the test.

The nurse quieted me down, and told me that they had completed all the necessary chest and liver area scans and only the head was not done, so the test was acceptable for my purposes. The test results did confirm my three liver tumors. When I repeated the PET scan at that same site a year later, they had changed the procedure so that your hands were above your head and not wrapped around your sides. The nurse told me that the change was due to patient feedback. I handled it much better the second time around.

STARTING CHEMO WITH THE HOME-MADE IV POLE: FEBRUARY 2004

The following Monday, my right arm chemo port was inserted. The insertion involves putting a tube into a deep vein in your arm that empties into the large vein in the chest. There is a port on the underside of the arm that provides easy access for chemo infusion, and also, I found, for drawing blood. And on Wednesday I reported to the chemo room at the local hospital for my first chemo session. The hospital chemo room was very nice, with soft leather chairs, about a dozen in all, and a lot of TV sets scattered around. The chemo program I was on was to take three consecutive days.

I found out that the procedures over the three days varied by the organization that was administrating them. At the hospital, the first day I had a pre-chemo steroid solution, followed by a two hour mix of Leucovorin and Oxaliplatin. I was then fitted out with a 24-hour, 5FU heavy brick-sized pump that was affixed to my waist, and I was sent home for the day. The next day, a home care nurse came to our house to clean the pump, administer two hours of Leucovorin and reload the pump for another 24 hour treatment. On the last day, she came to the house to clean up the stuff, and I was free for the next two weeks until we were to start the process all over again.

One interesting point regarding my first home treatment was the necessity of finding something that could serve as an "IV" pole for the chemo. The nurse and I looked around the downstairs of my home and eventually we settled on an antique clothes pole that Pat and I had purchased while we lived in Europe and used in the front hall as a coat rack. You can imagine Pat's surprise when she returned home that Thursday morning in February to find me sitting in a chair in our living room with the clothes pole serving as a chemo pole for my home treatment. By the way, trying to sleep with that big pump on my waist was next to impossible.

By the time I had my next chemo treatment two weeks later, Dr. Yi had received approval to administer Oxaliplatin. The treatment was done at Dr. Yi's infusion room and the experience was a lot different. The first day was basically the same, but at the end of the session, rather than being fitted out with a large waist pump, they taped a small heat activated pump device onto my arm near my port and attached a small bottle, (not unlike a baby bottle,) to the pump. I then threaded the cord connecting the device through my shirt sleeve so I could put the bottle in my shirt pocket.

I learned that the "baby bottle" is called a Baxter bottle. The heat pump would infuse the 5FU in the bottle for the next 22 hours or until the bottle was empty. After which, instead of having a nurse come to the house, I would return to the chemo room when the bottle was empty and have the next day's treatment. This was a much more civilized approach and a better use of time than the approach used at the hospital. I just had to watch the bottle, and go to the chemo room when it was empty. I also found that with the bottle I had a lot more freedom. I could drive more easily; go to the office, etc. The only thing that I did not do was sleep. Not because of the bottle but because of the steroids that they gave me with the chemo. I learned that for the first night of chemo and maybe the second, I would not get much, if any, sleep.

I have been told that having chemo is like having an individual clinical trial. No two people react the same way to a given chemo treatment. And I found that I might have different reactions to the same chemo program at different times. I was able to tolerate the dosage of the FOLFOX 4 that I was given, although I learned from the chemo nurses that a number of people were not able to tolerate the side effects and had to either reduce the dosage or eliminate some of the treatment altogether.

One of the early side effects of Oxaliplatin was the intolerance to cold. It comes on almost immediately after your first course of treatment. I could not touch anything cold: the refrigerator door, the mail box in winter, maybe the front door handle, the car door, without getting a kind of shock. The shock was somewhat similar to that you might get from a jolt of static electricity. I found it helpful to leave a pair of gloves on the kitchen counter and put them on if I was going to open the refrigerator. I also kept an extra pair of gloves upstairs and often slept with them on. Very romantic.

I also could not drink anything cold, particularly if it had ice cubes in it. If I made the mistake of drinking ice water, I would get sharp pains in the back of my mouth like you might get if you swallowed some razor blades. You quickly learned what you could do and not do. You also lose your taste buds so most of your food tastes quite bland.

You learn to appreciate the chemo nurses. At the time, in Dr. Yi's chemo room there were Barbara, Lori, Amy & Joan. They have a really tough job. Probably no patient in the chemo room wants to be there, but everyone knows that you have to go through it if you are going to have a chance. The nurses approach everyone with dignity and professionalism. And while they cannot tell you specifics about individual patients, they can tell you a lot about the specific treatment that you are having and help you to know what to expect. Sometimes there are doughnuts or cookies available and when you "graduate," or have your last treatment, they sprinkle you with magic dust to help you on your road to recovery.

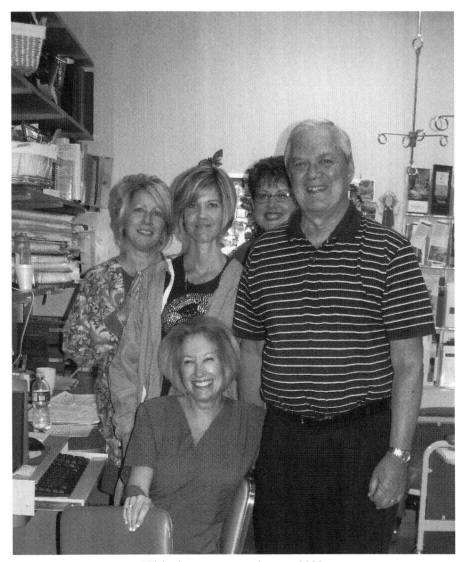

With chemo nurses- August 2009

THE DVT

You have to watch the various reactions that your body has to the treatments. Probably the worst was just before my third chemo treatment when I noticed some swelling in my port arm. When I met with Dr. Yi that day, rather than send me to the chemo room for treatment, he ordered an ultrasound test done on the arm but didn't tell me what was wrong. I asked the ultrasound nurse if the test showed anything wrong. She said "I can't tell you that. But I can say that you were lucky not to have had chemo today."

When I returned to his office, Dr. Yi said that I had a DVT (Deep Vein Thrombosis) or blood clot in my port arm and he was sending me directly to the hospital. I said, "What?" And he said that he was writing an emergency order and I was to immediately check into the Medical Center. While I cheated a bit and went home first to leave a note for Pat about this diversion, I then went and checked into the hospital.

This was actually a very serious matter, for I learned that if the clot is released into the blood stream it could go to the lungs to cause pulmonary embolism. But they gave me injections to thin the blood to help dissolve the clot, adjusted my Coumadin dosage, and monitored me. In four days, the clot had cleared; it was no longer a problem and I was released.

It turned out to be a fairly civilized hospital experience. Since I was on the cancer floor, I had a private room. I was on a full diet the whole time. No catheter. No IV pole. And I actually slept in my pajamas. Fortunately, the problem never came back again, although I did spend a day in the emergency room about two weeks later when my whole upper body turned red without any obvious reason. After the day spent there, they finally released me and wrote it off as a chemo reaction.

I started to manage the treatments pretty well. You learn how to schedule your life around the chemo. I found out that it took my body about a week to recover after a chemo treatment. That meant that if I completed my treatment on a Thursday, by the following Wed or so I was feeling reasonably civilized again and my bodily functions may be somewhat back to normal. If Pat and I wanted to plan a dinner out with friends, go to a concert, or something like that we would do it on the off weekend, knowing that on the weekend just following the chemo I would not be in good shape.

Also I learned that I could not plan much for the evenings during the chemo sessions. Once I tried to go to choir practice on a Wed evening just after chemo and I found that I was very tired and not much good at practice. Dr. Yi said that I should just stay home and rest during those times. So it was basically one week on and one week off, a process that was continued over most of the next five years.

CHAPTER 7:
Am I Going to Die?

I think one of the first questions cancer patients ask themselves is "Is it going to get me? Am I going to die?" In the early phase of your treatment you don't know what to expect. You don't know if the chemo is going to work. You have read so many bad reports about cancer that you can easily get discouraged. And you start having talks with your spouse about what would happen if you were gone.

I had several friends that I sang with in the bass section of our church choir that had different cancers and were not doing well, so you see the results of cancer all around you. But you realize that neither you nor your doctors know exactly what will happen in your specific case. All you can do is to follow the plan that you and they have laid out and hope for the best.

And I developed the attitude that if I was feeling reasonable well, then the cancer could not be doing too much damage. So as long as I felt well I felt that I must be ok and had hope. And you also know that life can be fickle and something other than cancer could strike you at any time. So the reality check is that the best you can do is to develop a plan and stick to it. *(See Lessons 3 & 6)*

The good news about my chemo program was that it worked. When I had scans at the end of three months, two of the spots in my right liver were gone and the one in my left liver had shrunk to about half of its original size. I was on the right track and we were very pleased with the results so far.

But it was beginning to look like I would need liver surgery to address the remaining spot in the left side of the liver, so it was time to visit Dr. Fong at MSKCC in NYC. At the time Pat and I were not too keen about having surgery in New York as opposed to some place more local in New Jersey, but we made the appointment and went to NYC to meet with Dr. Fong. That turned out to be one of the more important decisions that we would make. He turned out to be both competent and confident. When Pat mentioned that we were all the way from Princeton, NJ, he commented that he had a patient down the hall from the Middle East, and that he considered Princeton to be local.

He said that the one remaining tumor in my left liver was operable, and that if the remaining chemo treatments did not shrink it any further, he would recommend surgery as soon as we could schedule it. He then gave us a little discussion on what the surgery would entail. I was not eager to have another surgery but we were glad that we had made contact with him and waited to see what the remaining chemo treatments would bring.

CHAPTER 8:
Family Time and Neuropathy

My daughter, Kelly, had been married in a small civil ceremony in England in September 2003. We wanted to have a US ceremony for her as well and had it scheduled for May 2004 at a nearby British type location called Fernbrook. One of my objectives with Dr. Yi was that I wanted to be able to schedule my chemo so that I could not only attend the ceremony, but walk Kelly down the aisle and dance the first dance with her. And I was able to do all of that.

It turned out to be a great international party. We had people there from all over: the Brits, Kelly's friends from when we lived in Hong Kong, her Georgetown classmates, NYC colleagues and Princeton friends, and our family and friends. I believe that the only problem I had was my hair did not cooperate and was kind of frizzy all day. It was a hot day and it may have been the humidity and not the chemo that affected my hair. I believe that one reason all of Pat's and my family members attended was not just to congratulate Kelly & Lewis, but also to see how I was doing.

On the evening before the party Pat and I hosted a barbeque reception at our home for our family members, Lewis's family, and some of the international travelers. One guest was Tara Butler, one of Kelly's best friends from the Hong Kong International School days when I worked for IBM in Hong Kong. She was living in Paris at the time and I remember spending time talking to her about her life there and wondering if I would ever be able to travel abroad again, let alone get back to Paris.

I had really enjoyed my international assignments and the excitement of overseas travel. I was bitten by the travel bug early in my life and was very lucky to have had opportunities to take advantage of it. I had first traveled overseas as a midshipman in the NROTC on cruises on the USS Missouri and USS Wisconsin, spent five months in the Mediterranean with the Navy, then toured Europe with the University of Michigan Men's Glee Club and followed that up with business trips with IBM, vacations in the Bahamas, the Caribbean and Mexico and IBM assignments in The Netherlands, Paris and Hong Kong. The thought of not being able to travel overseas again because of concerns about chemo treatments or hospitals was a real damper on my enthusiasm, but there was not much I could do about it at the time, except do the best I could with the program that I was on.

(It has nothing to do with cancer, but I would like to mention that the University of Michigan Men's Glee Club is celebrating its 150th anniversary in 2009, and it is also the 50th anniversary of the club winning first prize in the International Musical Eisteddfod in Llangollen, Wales, the first American glee club to do so. I sang with the club for three years and was fortunate to have participated in that event.)

NEUROPATHY – SUMMER 2004

I completed 12 rounds of chemo in mid-July and had a set of scans and another colonoscopy. The colonoscopy was normal, but, whereas I was hoping that the scans would show further reduction in the remaining liver spot, they did not. The chemo response had plateaued and the spot was about the same size it had been in April. We now had to discuss our next steps and the proposed liver surgery. It was a disappointment but not the end of the world.

We decided to go back to the Cancer Institute of New Jersey to get an opinion from Dr. Poplin, the colon cancer oncologist that I had met back in January. Taking my latest sets of scans, Pat & I drove up to the New Brunswick facility. Dr. Poplin thought that I had done very well on the first six months of chemo and appeared to have tolerated it better than most patients do.

But when I tried to button my shirt I had difficulty in sensing the buttons. She said, "It looks like you have neuropathy." I said "What is that? She said that I was in the early stages of peripheral neuropathy, which is damage to the nerve endings in the hands and feet caused by the toxicity of Oxaliplatin. Since I had already completed 12 courses of FOLFOX 4, Dr. Poplin said that she would recommend to Dr Yi that I stop the Oxaliplatin immediately, and continue on with just Leucovorin and 5FU until we made a decision on the surgery. When we had our appointment with Dr. Yi the following week, he said that he had talked to Dr. Poplin and concurred with the recommendation.

The neuropathy started in my hands and then moved to my feet. I could not sense anything in my fingertips. I could not type at a computer without hunting and pecking with the keys. I could not pick up paper clips, pens or pencils without looking at them. I could not feel the change in my pocket. I could not feel a coffee cup in my right hand. To hold a cup I had to put my left hand underneath the cup to keep it from falling. I had difficulty turning the pages of a book or a music score.

It was quite discouraging. Walking upstairs and downstairs became more of a chore. I had to take it very slow and easy, but I could manage. With neuropathy you do not have normal feeling in the front of your feet from the instep to your toes. It's kind of like walking on a bed of uneven sponges or rags. Walking upstairs I did not have a feel for the steps. And walking downstairs I had to learn to balance on my heels which is not normal, but it works. The feeling in your feet goes from tingling to numbness.

Walking barefoot on grass or a driveway would feel like walking on coals or nails. And after walking a distance in your shoes, your feet could bind up. It makes things like driving a car more difficult. And you can't stand for any long periods of time. If I had to stand, I tried to find something to lean against so that I could balance on the heels of my feet.

I tried acupuncture for several months to see if that would help but it didn't seem to make any difference. I was told that I could expect the neuropathy to go away over time. But I have since been to see a neurologist and he has told me that if the normal feeling in my feet and hands had not come back in three years, it was unlikely to do so. So I am left with it. But in the grand scheme of things, if I traded two eliminated and one shrunk cancer tumors for neuropathy, it is not a bad trade-off.

I have since learned that FOLFOX with Oxaliplatin is still the first line treatment for advanced colon cancer even though many patients get neuropathy. They have tried to give pre-chemo doses of calcium and magnesium to offset the problem, but nothing seems to work. So the neuropathy will probably continue to be a by-product of colon cancer chemo for the time being.

We are fortunate enough to have a backyard pool; we have had one since 1984, and one thing that I enjoy in the summer is swimming. And other than using a service to open and close the pool, I normally take care of checking the chemicals, cleaning out the skimmer, etc and otherwise maintaining it in swimming condition.

Imagine my surprise when I put my hand into the skimmer to clean out the debris and got a bit of a shock. And then I tried to put my foot into the pool to test my ability to swim. No way. The neuropathy made it too uncomfortable. So while I did my best to keep the chemicals up to snuff, I was not able to swim at all during the summer of 2004. It was very disappointing.

Also I could not button or unbutton my shirts. The worst thing was buttoning shirt sleeves, which I would normally do with one hand but now could not manage at all. So for the next six months Pat had to button up my shirts in the morning and unbutton them for me at night. It became a daily ritual. I was also worried about how I was going to be able to hold my new grandchild in December. And I found out later that due to the neuropathy, I would no longer be able to wiggle my ears for my grandchildren. But that is all getting ahead of the game.

CHAPTER 9:
Memorial Sloan Kettering Cancer Center

The next step was to see Dr. Fong again and schedule the liver surgery. We had consulted with Dr. Yi and determined that while the chemo might slow the cancer down, the only way to get rid of the tumor in the left side of the liver and go for a cure was surgery. So we made the appointment to see Dr. Fong in NYC. By this time our daughter, Kelly, had a job with ESPN in NYC and was living there, so we were able to combine a doctor's visit with a lunch with her.

We started trying to make the NYC trips a family visit with a side trip to the doctor instead of the other way around. That way they became a fun day in NYC, although I was frequently carrying films under my arm during the day. In any case, Dr. Fong wanted to schedule the surgery as soon as possible. I had to be off chemo for a month before the surgery so we had to coordinate the surgery date with Dr. Yi. We had a vacation planned at our time share in Longboat Key, Florida in the middle of October and we needed time for the pre-admission testing. So we scheduled this surgery for October 26, 2004 at Memorial Sloan Kettering Hospital on York Ave in NYC.

———————

We were searching for as much information on colon cancer that we could find. There was not an official colon cancer support group in the Princeton area, so I tried to find out as much as I could from informal sources. There was a Cancer Care counselor who came to Princeton once a week. Pat and I met with her to get any information that she might have. I also got several phone numbers for cancer survivors around the country.

In September we went to an anniversary party for one of our neighbors and met a colon cancer patient there who had had the liver surgery and needed to have a liver chemo pump installed. It had not gone well for him and I vowed to avoid a liver pump if at all possible. You learned quite a bit by talking to people who had been down the path.

Pat & I also talked to a number of people in the Princeton area who, while they did not have colon cancer, had been successful with other cancers. There were several people from our Coldwell Banker office who had had successful outcomes working with Dr. Yi. Dr. Lyn Ransom, the founder and music director of the Voices Chorale, was diagnosed with breast cancer shortly after my colon cancer diagnosis. She has recovered well and I continue to be impressed with her energy and enthusiasm in directing Voices rehearsals and concerts. I don't know how she is able to stand for such long periods of time. I guess that if you are going to be a choir conductor, it comes with the territory.

Two of my fellow basses in Voices have had bouts with prostate cancer and seem to be doing quite well. And Stuart Pope, a bass member of our church choir and a past president of the Voices Chorale, had fought cancer for over 12 years before passing away in early 2005. I would often see him and his wife in Dr. Yi's offices. He was singing and playing the church organ up until the end of 2004, and he continues to be a strong inspiration for me.

We were also getting a lot of requests from family and friends for updates on my progress. So we set up three layers of email lists; first to our immediate family including our son Scott, his wife Cristina, and our daughter, Kelly. The second list was to both Pat's and my brothers and sisters. When we started this journey, she had two living brothers who were on our list. I have four brothers and a sister. So that was the second list we used. And thirdly there were the various friends and business associates who wanted to be updated. Frequently we would get calls or emails from friends who had heard about my situation and wanted to be included. That list continued to grow over the course of my treatments and currently has about 50 names on it.

Over the six years we have received innumerable emails, encouraging cards, calls of support and visits from these family members and friends. Next to the caregiver, I feel having a reliable network of family and friends is a very important part of dealing with the cancer experience. *(See Lesson 7)*

After an abbreviated vacation at the timeshare on Longboat Key, we returned to have my pre-admission testing done in NYC. Everything went well and I was good to go for surgery the following week. One pre-admission test I had done before the Florida trip was a stress test by the heart specialist that I had met in the hospital in Princeton and that test was fine. Dr. Fong just wanted to make sure that my heart was ok before operating on my liver.

My daughter, Kelly, offered to have Pat stay with her at her NYC apartment during my hospital stay. This worked out extremely well since her apartment was on Lexington Avenue only about six blocks from the hospital. A neighbor and fellow church member, John Powell, had agreed to drive us up to the hospital for my 5:30 AM check-in for the surgery. So all was set.

About 4:00 in the morning on Oct 26 we left 43 Beech Hill Circle for NYC and the Memorial Sloan Kettering Hospital on York Ave on the East Side. We arrived in plenty of time for my check-in and prep time. It turned out that John Powell had spent a summer as a cab driver in Chicago, so the NYC driving was no problem for him. I was to be Dr. Fong's first surgery that day.

We learned that he operates primarily on Tuesday and Thursday, two surgeries a day. On Monday he has office hours; on Wednesday and Friday he catches up on the surgeries that he might have as emergency cases. All told he does well over 200 surgeries a year, all either liver or stomach related cancer operations, probably more than any other surgeon in the US. When we had questioned Dr. Fong about the problems we had read about concerning blood loss in liver surgery, his comment was, "Not on my watch."

My wife continues to be impressed with the treatment that patients get at MSKCC. At the doctors' offices they have someone to meet you at the door to make sure you know how to get to the right place. At the hospital they take special care of the patients checking in for surgery. They obviously know that anyone that shows up at their door is there because they have something serious going on in their bodies and they want to do their best to make people feel at ease and comfortable. Pat particularly has remarked about the live orchids that they have in the doctor's waiting room.

As far as I know the first liver surgery was pretty straightforward. Dr. Fong made a straight vertical cut to line up with my colon scar. Then he took out one section of the left side of my liver, checked out the location of the original two spots on the right side of my liver and looked around to see any additional traces of cancer. Found nothing. Then he stapled me up.

I have since learned that the liver has eight sections; four on the left and four on the right. When you take out a section of the liver, it does not grow back but the remaining sections enlarge to fill in for the missing section. So in effect you end up with as much liver as you started with, only fewer sections.

I woke up in the recovery room which was quite different than the recovery room at the University Medical Center at Princeton. As memory serves me, this was a large room with monitor screens all around. Each patient that had been operated on that day (and I think that they had upwards of 15 operating rooms, with maybe 2 operations each) was in a separate curtained-off space in the large room. There was a control facility in the center of the room. Each patient had monitoring equipment connected up to the control facility.

And you spent the night there instead of being moved immediately to a hospital room.

My wife, son, Scott, and daughter, Kelly, all were there for my first NYC surgery. It was a stressful situation for all of us. One of the things that Pat remembered most about the whole Sloan Kettering experience was the intensity of the atmosphere in the recovery room. She said that it reminded her of the CTU set in the TV show "24".

Around mid-morning the next day, someone came in and announced the room assignments and you were rolled off to the hospital room where you would spend the rest of your stay. They probably found over time, and with the type of surgeries that they were doing, that the central controlled recovery space was a more efficient way to do it and had better results for the patients.

My first stay at Sloan Kettering was somewhat uneventful. I remember my first day in the hospital room with all of the supporting paraphernalia: vibrating booties, catheter, IV drip, pain medicine apparatus, as well as the ball apparatus to suck up to test your lungs and the iced swabs to suck on in lieu of water. And, of course, my "hug-me" pillow that we had brought from Princeton.

As soon as I could, I started questioning the doctors about how soon I could get out. Their original prognosis was a seven to ten day hospital stay. The first thing I had to be able to do was to swing my-self up and out of bed. That involved twisting my lower body so my feet would be over the side of the bed and then swinging my upper body up so that I was in a sitting position. And from there I would move down to a stand up position so that I could walk. The first day in the room, they had me up and walking around the nurse's station, although I was a bit slow and required someone to help hold me.

Since Pat was staying at Kelly's apartment on Lexington Ave, she would come to the hospital every morning to be with me, and help me on my walks. By day three, I was up and about on my own. I believe they told me that when I could do fifteen rounds around the floor I was a candidate to be released, so I worked on that objective. In any case, I got released in six days. Not that I was trying to set any kind of record, but I felt that I could recover better at home where I was not getting poked and prodded every few hours.

The one thing that I remember about that first visit to MSKCC was my roommate. He was from Long Island and would get phone calls and visitors at odd times of the day. During most of the phone calls he would say things in a low Godfather-like voice such as, "Thank you for that information," and "I am so glad that you brought that to my attention," etc . And when people came to visit they would always talk in hushed tones. Most of his visitors came late in the evening. I thought that he might be a member of the Mafia and was continuing to conduct his business from his hospital bed. Only in NYC.

Once home from that surgery, I recovered pretty quickly. I did go back on chemo for three months for what is called adjuvant therapy, but that was uneventful. When Pat & I went back to see Dr. Fong for a follow-up visit and to have my staples removed, he was very pleased with my progress and said: "I hope that you never have to see me again," meaning that he hoped that I was cured. And I hoped so as well. Then Pat and I went out for lunch in NYC to celebrate.

CHAPTER 10:
A Look Back At Pre-cancer Days

Thinking back to the start of all of this in pre-cancer days, I remember that at the beginning of 2003 things were looking good for the Cooke family. My wife and I were in good health, or so we thought, and looking forward to celebrating our 35th wedding anniversary that year.

We had two healthy children who had graduated from reputable schools, Colgate and Georgetown. The previous year, our son, Scott, had married a wonderful, talented girl, Cristina Egge, from Arlington, Virginia, whom he met at Graduate school at the University of Michigan. Her mother is originally from Madrid, Spain so the ceremony was held at a church in downtown Madrid and the reception at a castle just outside of town.

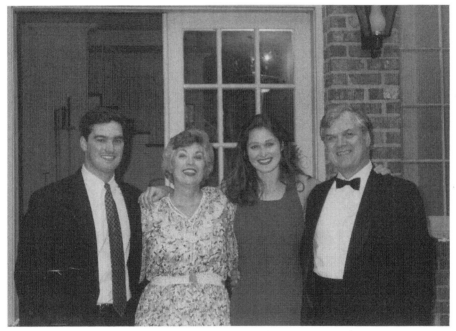

Kelly's Graduation at Georgetown –June 1994

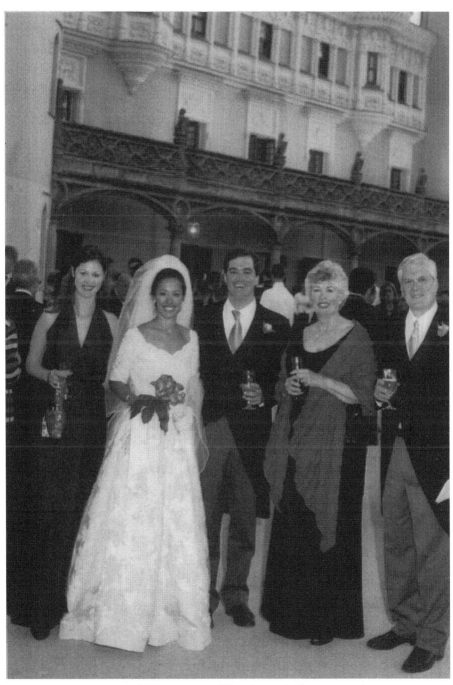

Scott and Cristina's Wedding in Madrid- June 2002

Our daughter, Kelly, was dating Lewis Reece, a tall, handsome Brit from Chipping Sodbury, England, whom she had met in Hong Kong. Since both Scott and Kelly had lived overseas for a good part of their lives, overseas travel came naturally to them, as well as to Pat and me.

So life was good. I had completed a successful career with IBM that had taken me from Jackson, Michigan to Detroit, to Pittsburgh, to Princeton, to Holland, to Paris, back to Princeton, to Hong Kong and then to an early retirement. Since 1995 I had been working with my wife in Real Estate in the Coldwell Banker Princeton office where she was one of the top agents. We had a nice home in Princeton Township, and a 1 year old collie named Luke.

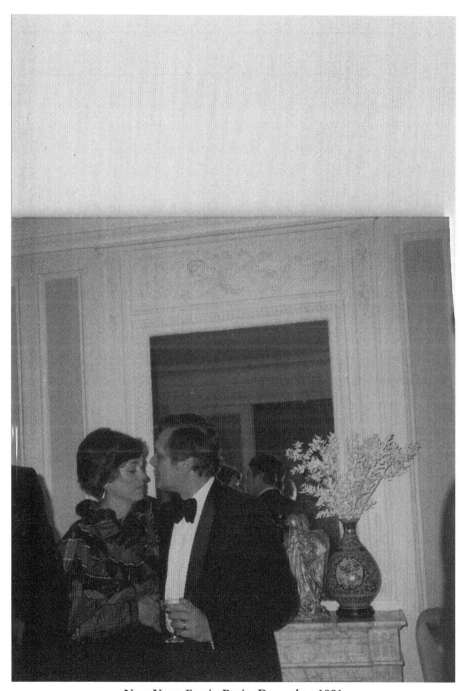

New Years Eve in Paris- December 1981

I had been active in several organizations. I had been instrumental in getting a scholarship in memory of my parents set up at Bowling Green State University in Ohio where my father had been a professor for years. Many BGSU people and my siblings have donated to it over the years and I believe that it is currently the largest non-corporate scholarship in the business school there. I had spent ten years on the Board of Trustees at my church and had been on the capital funds and building committees for the major renovation and building of a second story addition to the church education building. As a result of our stock gifts to the capital funds drive, Pat and I were eligible to have one of the newly renovated classrooms dedicated to the memory of our parents.

I have had a number of memorable experiences over my life like singing in Carnegie Hall and spending eight years with my wife and family living and working overseas with IBM in three countries. But the 40 year success of our marriage, and helping Pat raise two intelligent, educated, talented and capable children, along with the setting up of the BGSU scholarship, and the renovation of the education building at the Princeton United Methodist Church with the church classroom dedicated to our parents, have got to be four of the proudest accomplishments of my life.

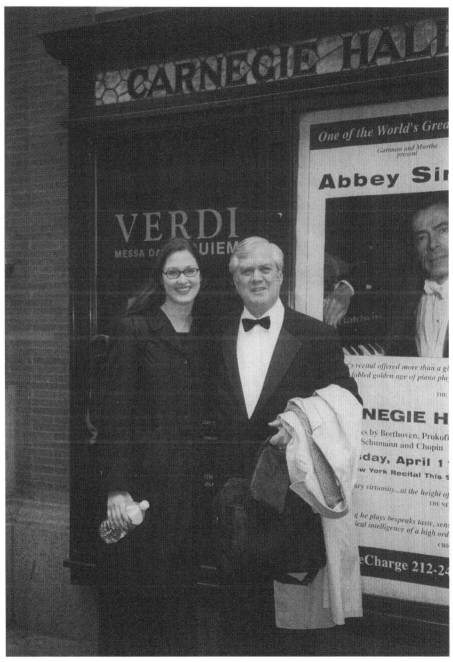

With Kelly after singing together in Carnegie Hall, November 2001

In 2003 Pat had qualified for a Coldwell Banker expense paid trip to the Breakers Hotel in Florida. And I tagged along. We were going back to Europe in May with the Voices Chorale to sing in Bavaria and Austria. And we were also planning to travel to our timeshare at Longboat Key in Florida in October and to Hilton Head in December for a reunion with Pat's family. I went to my doctor only once or twice a year to check out normal stuff like cholesterol, blood pressure and PSA. I may have been a bit overly optimistic about how well things were going for us. It was a busy and exciting life.

Then we got hit with cancer. It was a bolt out of the blue. Getting hit with cancer changes how you look at things. It scares you. As I mentioned previously, it makes you question your mortality. And you start to think about how the life of the people around you would be impacted if you were not there. But you then realize that you could just as easily get hit by a car or something else, so life is fragile and you shouldn't focus too much on that problem. Then, it made us aware of the number of people that we knew who were facing difficult illnesses. As we started to inform people of my situation, we became knowledgeable of many other people who were dealing with or had dealt with potentially life threatening diseases. I have already mentioned a few of them. And it makes you appreciate what they are going through all the more.

It also makes you aware of the high cost of cancer treatment. I was fortunate to have Medicare and a supplemental retiree medical plan from IBM, although they are increasingly asking retirees to shoulder a larger cost of the plan. But if you look at the gross cost of a single week of chemo treatment, it can make you shudder.

In any case, getting hit with cancer makes you appreciate more the days that you have.

Now I try to get the most that I can out of every day. I keep lists of things to do and try to focus on the most important things, for the day, the week, the month, the rest of the year, and even the next five years.

I am hopeful that I will be able to keep going for a long time. I want to make the best of the remainder of my life and also make the best of my time with my wife, family and friends. I don't want to look back when and if they tell me that the cancer can no longer be treated, which could very well happen some day, and find something that I could have done and didn't. *(See Lesson 14)* I also want to do what I can to help others who are dealing with cancer learn and benefit from my experiences.

CHAPTER 11:
Your Mind And Your Body

My son, Scott, and his wife, Cristina, were expecting their first child, and our first grandchild, in December 2004. Pat arranged a baby shower at the Nassau Club in Princeton. It is a dining club in downtown Princeton that we have been members of for about ten years. My brother, Jim, and his wife, Janet, came over from Philadelphia for the day- Janet to join the ladies at the baby shower, and Jim to talk to me at home while I recuperated from my October surgery.

Jim has been suffering from Parkinson's and has all of the normal symptoms; difficulty talking, some palsy, and in general a slower pace. He first noticed the symptoms around 2000 and was diagnosed with the disease in 2002. He discussed with me a concept that I had not thought about before; which is, that while he may have physical difficulties with his body, he still had control over his mind. And he found comfort in separating his still intact vibrant mind from his physical being. We talked about that concept for the better part of the afternoon while the ladies were out.

I have thought about that concept a lot over the past five years and truly believe that if we focus on the things that we can do, particularly with our minds, that it can help balance out the problems that we may have with our bodies. We may not have any say in the diseases that we may have, whether it is Parkinson's, cancer or something else, but we do have a say in how we respond to them. *(See Lesson 8)*

And on December 12, 2004 our first grandchild, Xavier, was born to our son, Scott, and his wife, Cristina. It was such a joyful event in the midst of everything else that was going on around us. I was afraid to hold him since my hands were still suffering from neuropathy and I was worried that I might drop him, but I solved the problem by wearing gloves.

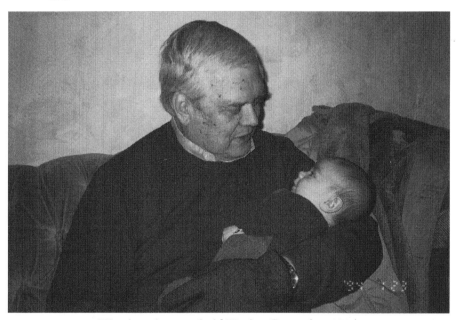

Wearing gloves to hold Xavier- December 2004

CHAPTER 12:
Growing Up In Bowling Green, Ohio

2005 was a pretty good year. I wrapped up my chemo treatments in February and started to live life as normal. Pat and I went to the Coldwell Banker International Business Conference in Orlando in February, a recognition event for the top performers of the previous year. I got back to singing in Voices where I had missed most of 2004 and I was able to sing in the performances of Handel's Saul and Beethoven's 9th. I also went to Carnegie Hall to hear Kelly sing in the Verdi Requiem; then to Savannah to Pat's brother's daughter, Jessica's wedding.

We had the dedication of the Methodist Church Education Building, a project that I had worked on for about eight years. I also joined a bible study group that met Thursday noon at our church. It was primarily men, but there were a couple of women there as well and it became an excellent support group for me. In between all of this I was seeing Dr. Yi and having scans. Everything was normal. I was beginning to have the feeling that I was cured.

That summer I could swim in the pool again. We got caught up with friends and in September went to California for the wedding of my Brother Jim's daughter, Josie, at Yosemite, followed by another set of normal scans and then a two week trip to Longboat Key in October. We finally decided in November to have my port removed so I would not have to put up with having it flushed once a month, taking Coumadin to thin my blood, and worrying about having another DVT.

Our real estate business was going along as well as could be expected, and, that November, I sang in Carnegie Hall again with Voices. I was keeping up pretty well. I told the minister at my church that I would be willing to serve on a couple of church committees. I had been quite active at the church until my original cancer diagnosis and felt that I once again had the ability to use my talents to serve in that capacity. Life was pretty good again, and I was feeling good and perhaps somewhat overly optimistic about the whole process.

I have had people tell me that they are amazed about my positive attitude through the whole cancer experience. I tell them that, while I appreciate their comment, it is just the way that I am. I am not trying to do anything special because of cancer; just acting normal for me. As I have thought more about that trait, I believe that it is something that I acquired as a child growing up in Bowling Green, Ohio. *(See Lesson 9)*

It was an idyllic existence. At the time, Bowling Green was a small town of about 14,000 people in the Northwestern part of Ohio with none of the disturbing things that you read today about kids growing up. At least none that I knew about. My father, Gilbert, was a college professor of business administration at the local University, BGSU. My mother, Lottie, was the daughter of a Minnesota farmer and a stay-at-home mom. And they had six kids, five boys and a girl; Dean, Wayne, Janet, Allen, Dan, and Jim. We were a fairly close-knit family.

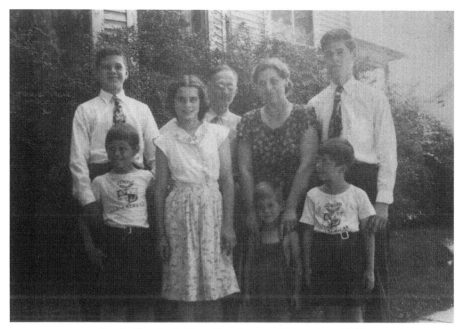

Cooke family in Bowling Green, Ohio, circa 1948

One of my memories of an event that impacted my early development came when I was about twelve years old. Mom had sent me to the Kroger store, about five blocks away, to pick up some groceries, which I remember included celery and a bag of sugar. Since it was during the rationing time of World War II, she had equipped me with the necessary ration stamps for the bag of sugar as well as money for the purchases.

I remember walking to the Kroger store, where my older brother, Dean, and I would later work during high school; bagging groceries and stocking shelves. I recall getting the groceries and coming home, whistling and happy about having successfully done my chore. I was not focusing at all on the grocery bag. Then when I got home, all hell broke loose.

The wet celery and the bag of sugar had come together in the grocery bag opening a hole through which about half of the sugar had spilled out somewhere along the sidewalk during my walk. My dad was livid. I had carelessly lost half of a month's ration of sugar. While my mother was understanding about the situation, as she normally was, Dad proceeded to lecture me on my perceived lackadaisical attitude. Whether rightly or wrongly, he wanted me to get the message that he thought I had messed up and he wanted to make it a learning experience. Pay attention to what you are doing. He made an impression on me that I obviously remember to this day.

He was also a firm believer in the value of education as well as the need to always use the skills that you were given. He used to tell the story of the two students: both got Bs on an exam. But they were not the same. One student was a C level student, so his (or her) B grade was an excellent performance for him (or her). The other was an A level student so his (or her) B grade was a wasted performance. The message of the parable: use your skills- don't waste them. And he strongly imparted those values to his six children, five of whom ended up with advanced degrees. He didn't have to say much. Just a few words and maybe the look on his face were all that it took to show either his pleasure or his displeasure with your performance.

I think that my siblings and I spent a good part of our early lives seeking acceptance from our father. And maybe that search for acceptance helped established a positive attitude in each of us. I learned that whether it is carrying groceries home from the store, studying to get good grades, or fighting cancer, you should always do the best you can with the skills that you have.

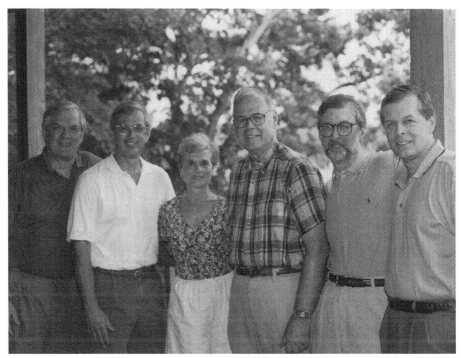

Wayne, Allen, Janet, Dean, Jim and Dan at family reunion, July 1999

THE BOTCHED BUGLER

Another childhood memory stands out as well. I learned at an early age that I was not a particularly good athlete. I remember that in the 8th grade when I tried out for football, I was 4'10" tall and weighed 88 lbs. This was not quite big enough to make it at football or basketball. So I focused my energy on my studies and on extra-curricular activities such as choir, student council, honor society, drama club, etc. I also learned how to play the ukulele. Outside of school I was a Cub Scout and then a Boy Scout and enjoyed going to the area scout camp, Camp Miakonda, in the summers.

When I was 15, I had an opportunity to work at the camp for the summer. They had only a few positions open and one was to be one of the two camp buglers. I had taken cornet lessons in elementary school, but had stopped in junior high. I had worked hard at the scout achievements, receiving the rank of Eagle Scout. Somewhere along the way, I had convinced someone that I qualified for the Bugler merit badge, so I appeared to be a good candidate for the camp staff.

After being selected, I attended a pre-camp orientation week for the new staff members. The other bugler and I were to alternate the playing duties during the week. These involved climbing the flag pole and playing reveille, morning flag ceremony, mess call three times a day, evening flag ceremony, and taps. Also fire call, if necessary.

After we had gone through several days of this, the staff counselor called me into his office. "Cooke," he said. "You are the worst bugler that we have ever had." I was devastated. It made no difference to him that just two weeks earlier I had received the American Legion Award as the outstanding boy graduating from Bowling Green Junior High School.

He had a more practical problem, which was helping run a scout camp. And he was probably right. I had been trying to get by on my reputation. I probably had not practiced as much as I should have and thought that I could get by, but when you are at the top of the flagpole with just yourself and the bugle, there is no place to hide. And since my father was the scoutmaster of our local scout troop and active in the area councils, getting sent home was not an alternative and I did not want to go through another talk with him.

Well, the net of the discussion that followed was that the staff counselor was going to talk to the other, more proficient bugler about taking over all of the bugling duties, and I was going to split my time between working in the camp store, The Trading Post, and serving as a lifeguard, all 115 lbs of me. I did have the swimming, lifesaving, rowing and canoeing merit badges so was actually pretty qualified in the aquatic stuff. (I had not applied for a lifesaving position in the first place because I was too small.)

He also wanted me to practice the bugle more in a cabin removed from the main camp-site so I would be ready in case of need. Back then they called it "wood shedding," So that's what I did. And at the end of the summer, the staff counselor called me back into his office to congratulate me on taking the reprimand and doing a commendable job in the alternative assignments. As my father would say, showing a little "gumption."

OFF THE FAMILY "PAYROLL"

I also came off of the Cooke Family "payroll" at a fairly early age by today's standards. I probably had an allowance as a kid although I can't remember how much it was. I had my first job, a paper route delivering the Toledo Blade, at around the age of eleven which helped pay for my candy bars, Saturday afternoon matinees at the local theater, collecting occasional stamps on approval and my comic books. (Whatever happened to my Superman comics is beyond me. I should have kept them.)

Then I got my first salaried job at the age of 15 working in a shoe repair shop for 25 cents per hour and opened my first savings account. At 16, I was able to step up to 65 cents per hour at the Kroger store, bagging groceries, stocking shelves and eventually working up to a check out cashier and produce clerk, which had a higher hourly rate. My senior year in high school, I was accepted for a Navy NROTC scholarship which paid my tuition, books and fees for my entire undergraduate education: the first two years in mathematics at The University of Missouri and the final two years at the Business School of the University of Michigan.

What with the money I had saved working at the Kroger store during high school and the food bills I avoided by washing pots and pans at a nearby sorority house, I believe that my cost to my parents for my entire college education was the sum total of $25 for a round trip train trip from Missouri to Ohio during a spring vacation. And with the money I had saved in the Navy and a part time job working in the Internal Audit Department of the University, I was able to pay for my Michigan MBA and took my $500 a month computer sales training job with IBM debt-free and ready to take on the world.

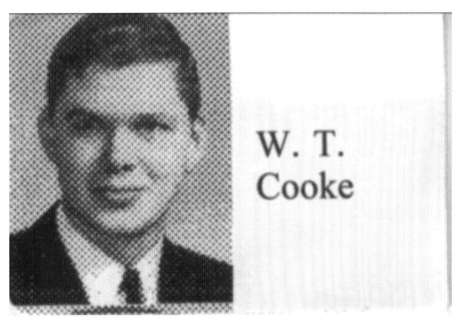

At University of Michigan, circa 1959

Hopefully the self sufficiency and positive attitude skills I learned then have also helped me to successfully take on my cancer. (*See Lesson 9*)

CHAPTER 13:
2006, Recurrence, Liver Surgery And Lung Spots

2006 changed things regarding my cancer recovery. I had claimed victory too soon. My scans the end of January showed a new spot on the right side of my liver. To say the least, it was a bummer. Dr. Yi had previously discussed with me the possibilities of a recurrence. He said that there was about a 50% chance that metastatic cancer could reappear. This was caused by microscopic spots that were originally too small to show up on scans, and after about 2-3 years they would finally be large enough to be seen. They were not new spots, but ones that had been there since the first metastasis and had survived the chemo attacks. It hit me totally by surprise. *(See Lesson 12)*

So back we went to NYC to see Dr. Fong. He confirmed that I had a spot on the right side of my liver, one that he had not seen when he had opened me up 15 months before. He said that he saw nothing else but the one spot and, since the previous chemo therapy had not worked on this spot, that the best solution for a cure was not additional chemo but to operate. We agreed and set the date for my next surgery for March 30, 2006.

I had a couple of things to get wrapped up. Pat and I were scheduled to go to San Francisco for the Coldwell Banker 100th Anniversary International Banking Conference. We did attend and saw a number of our California friends while there. Since my first liver surgery, Dr. Yi had put me on a one glass of wine a week limit. However, he agreed that while in California I could expand on that limit to taste some more California Sonoma Valley wines. And I did indeed.

We also saw Kelly sing at Carnegie Hall again. She was getting way ahead of me in Carnegie Hall appearances and, with my three lifetime appearances so far, I will probably never be able to catch up. There were also some Voices concerts in early March in Pennsylvania and Pennington where I wanted to sing and was able to do so. I could not stand for long periods of time without the neuropathy causing cramping in my feet, so I arranged with our director that I would sit while singing. I continually found singing to be a source of personal inner satisfaction, and my voice seemed to be holding up fairly well through all of this.

BACK TO MEMORIAL SLOAN KETTERING CANCER CENTER – MARCH 2006

We knew the drill at MSKCC, and the surgery and recovery were uneventful. This time the cut was an inverted L shape with the bottom of the L running horizontally across the right side of my stomach. The thing that made it interesting this time was again my roommate. He was apparently running a business from his hospital room.

I found out that he was a consultant to some non-profit organizations and did not want them to know that he was in the hospital. He had a private nurse running a phone setup so people that called in got him directly on his business phone number and would not know that he was hospitalized. He was taking calls all of the time. I finally asked one of the nurses why he was not in a private room. Maybe his medical plan did not cover it, although the nurse he had was there full time during the day and, I think, at his expense. In any case, by the end of my stay we were talking, and he turned out to be an interesting guy. He was actually a doctor who, in addition to the non-profit consulting business, was advising patients from his hospital bed. Very ingenious.

Pat, who was staying again at our daughter, Kelly's, apartment on Lexington Ave, would come to the hospital every morning and bring me the paper. She would stay with me in the room for the better part of the day, but I encouraged her to take the opportunity to see some museums if she had the chance. I looked forward to her arrival every day.

Kelly, who was working in NYC, was a frequent visitor to the hospital. According to her remembrance, when she took me on one of my early walks around the nurse's station, I was cruising the floor humming a tune from Star Wars. Scott, who works in Princeton, was able to visit on the weekend, and was responsible for bringing me my first Sudoku puzzle book. My brother, Jim and his wife, and my minister and his wife all came to NYC to visit with me at the hospital.

I spent much of my free time in the hospital working on the Sudoku puzzles. Dr. Fong would even give me daily puzzle completion objectives as part of my recovery procedures. I could do some fairly difficult ones but not the hardest. Today my brother, Allen, from Williamsburg, VA frequently sends me "evil" puzzles from WebSudoku that he claims he can solve in 20 minutes. I have difficulty solving them. I think he is subtly trying to prove to me that his MBA from Indiana University is better than mine from the University of Michigan. Again I made it out in six days. It was a very civilized hospital experience and I was in very good spirits when I left.

At home, spring was coming. I got my son, Scott, to help with the yard work and I was able to rest up out on the deck. By May, I was

able to sing in one of the Voices concerts, open the pool and go swimming. In June Pat and I took a trip to Tucson and then to Dallas for
the wedding of my Brother Dan's daughter, Gretchen. All seemed
well again.

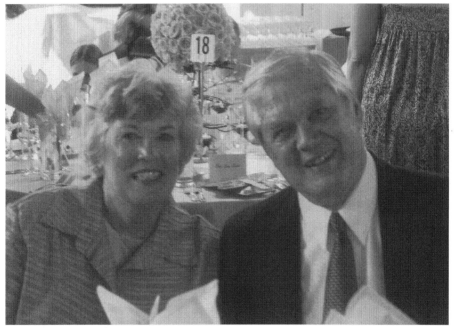

With Pat at Dallas wedding- June 2006

THE LUNGS- JULY 2006

Not so fast, Cooke. Just when things were looking good again,
my scans in July showed growth in both the number and size of pulmonary nodules in my lungs; on both the right and left sides of the
lungs to boot. PET scans confirmed the problems; and, to compound
matters, while I was having my PET scan, Pat fell at the doctors office and broke her ankle. We were back in the trenches again. We
could not seem to get ahead of the game. It was very frustrating.
(See Lesson 11)

I had a new arm port installed -left side this time- and went back on chemo. This was a new chemo regime called FOLFIRI plus Avastin. FOLFIRI is the familiar 5FU and Leucovorin plus a newer chemo called Irinotecan or Camptosar. Avastin is a new drug that is technically not chemo but is a monoclonal antibody that uses anti-angiogenic therapy to go after the blood supply of cancers. Irinotecan, I learned, causes you to lose your hair while the prior FOLFOX regime did not. So here we were.

I started chemo the first week of August, and by the end of August my hair started falling out in clumps. I also found out that I didn't need to shave as much as normal. But I figured that if the chemo caused me to lose my hair, it must also be creating problems for the cancer cells as well.

The chemo regime this time was a little better since they now used a forty-six hour Baxter bottle, twice the size of the former one. They had also eliminated the second day Leucovorin dosage. This meant that I did not have to go to the chemo room on the middle day of treatment, but just go around with my bottle. I bought a belt pack to stuff the bottle in and most people probably did not know that I was on chemo. I was tolerating the chemo but did have a number of different side effects from my first go-around in 2004. It intensified the neuropathy in my fingers and feet, and I had a lot more fatigue. Naps every afternoon.

THE GOOD DR. YI

I should comment that during the course of my journey, Dr. Yi is the doctor that I have seen the most. When I first went on chemo, I would see him every week; the first week to make sure that my blood counts were good enough to start the treatment that day, and the next week to see how my counts had reacted to the treatment. We have now cut that back to seeing him on the chemo weeks only. But if you figure that I was on chemo for most of 2004, and about half of 2006, 2007 and 2008, and infusional therapy for most of 2009 I must have seen Dr. Yi over 80 times. Pat has gone with me for many of those visits.

The routine is pretty much the same each time. I have blood drawn either at the lab or from my chemo port, and then see Dr. Yi after the blood results are back. He comes into the procedure room always smiling and upbeat. He reviews the results of my blood tests, and discusses my next treatment. He is always both professional and yet compassionate.

Pat and I will ask him any questions that we may have. No question is too stupid, simple or complex for him to give us his honest opinion. He also encourages us to get second opinions if we think them necessary. If I have just had scans or other tests, he reviews the test results and gives us his views on what they mean. And he is on top of his game. We trust him immensely and are very fortunate to have him available so near to us to advise us.

For his part, he must appreciate having a patient who is responding well to the treatments. Dr. Yi has two sons, one of whom sang at the American Boychoir School in Princeton, so he is very familiar with music, and often after we are through discussing cancer, he will ask about my singing experiences.

Dr. Yi is also supported by an excellent nurse staff. I have already mentioned the chemo room staff earlier in this journal. He also has an excellent primary nurse, Jean, who keeps track of everything. You know that you have been around a long time when you are on a first name basis with all of the nurses.

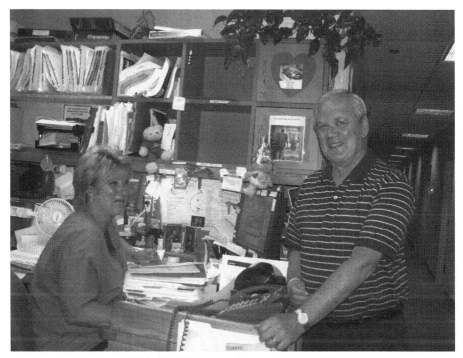

With Dr. Yi's nurse, Jean- August 2009

STAYING THE COURSE

After almost three years in the battle, our activities started to fit into a routine. I was determined that I wanted to be able to control my life and not let the cancer control me. In September 2006 we took time out to go to Ohio and Michigan for my high school reunion and visit old friends. And in Oct, Pat and I went back to Longboat Key for our annual R&R visit. But we were not sure what my long term prognosis was going to be. I did not seem to be able to keep ahead of the cancer. It was hard sometimes to remain positive. As my hair kept falling out, I started wearing hats, and have a collection now of various hats and caps. I guess the most important thing that I learned was to just take it a day at a time. *(See Lesson 13)*

Finally in November, we got some good news. My scans then showed the largest nodule in my lungs had shrunk to about half its original size; the second largest nodule had shrunk as well while the rest were unchanged. And there were no new nodules. Hurray! We would continue the chemo until I had been through 12 courses, which would take us through the middle of February 2007, have scans again and consider my next course of action.

I was continuing to sing as much as I could in both the church choir and the Voices Chorale. Voices was planning a trip to Germany/Italy in the spring of 2007 and I wanted to go if I could. I told Dr. Yi about it and he said that while singing was good for both my lungs and my mental health, he was not ready to approve me for an international trip just yet. He was concerned about what kind of medical care I might need in case of an emergency. We would monitor my condition, see how I progressed and hold off on a final decision regarding the trip until after the first of the year.

NEW CHALLENGES: THANKSGIVING- 2006

On the Monday after Thanksgiving we found out that our almost two- year-old grandson, Xavier, had acute lymphoblastic leukemia (ALL), which is the most common form of childhood cancer. And to complicate matters further, his parents, Scott and Cristina, were expecting their second child in March. Xavier prepared to start a six-month program of intensive treatment and chemo at the Morristown, NJ Children's Cancer Hospital, to be followed by a three-year maintenance program. Then on December 28th we learned that Pat's younger brother, Buzz, had died in a fire in their bed and breakfast inn in Franklin, NC, leaving behind his wife, Nancy, and three daughters. To put it mildly, Pat and I had more than our fair share of challenges to deal with.

CHAPTER 14:
2007, Treated But Not Cured

THE LOOK

2007 turned out to be a transition year from focus on surgery to focus on chemo treatments.

Pat and I occasionally went to an inexpensive family restaurant in nearby Montgomery, but had not been there since I had started this latest period of chemo. When we went in January, the assistant manager came over to say hello. We didn't know her by name but recognized her when we saw her. When she came over to our booth, I had already taken off my hat. She commented that she had not seen us for some time and then said that she thought that I had "the look." I knew what she was talking about since at that time I did not have much, if any, hair and was a little pasty from the chemo treatments. I tried to pass it off and to change the subject, saying that we had not been in for some time since I had been undergoing treatments. Pat later found out that her husband had been treated for cancer, so she was familiar with "the look." I vowed to do my best to get rid of it.

In February 2007, things for me started to improve. My scans showed the lung nodules were still stable, and sub-centimeter in size and, with recommendations by both Dr. Poplin and Dr. Yi, I started on an indefinite chemo holiday- and my hair started to come back.

Xavier completed his six-month intensive leukemia treatment program successfully in June 2007 and went on the three year maintenance program. He had lost his hair, and the steroids he was on caused some irritability and weight gain, but that is behind him now. As an aside, we have some interesting pictures of him and his grandpa when both of us were kind of bald. His hair came back in a youthful brush cut, and he was running around like a typical three year old. And he became a big brother. His sibling, Rafael, was born March 2, 2007 and is a delightful grandson.

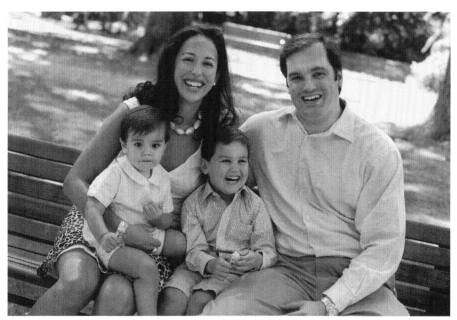

Scott, Cristina and the boys- December 2008

I continued on my chemo holiday in 2007, and was able to work on the church Endowment Fund committee. I was able to sing in two performances of Brahms Requiem and also to go on the Voices trip to Europe. I was worried about problems with my feet while standing for the concerts, so I took along a folding chair that worked out well for three of the Italian concerts. I also took along a cane which helped while walking the cobblestone streets and in particular going up and down the bridges in rainy Venice. The weather was not so good in Italy, but the singing was excellent. I was glad that I was able to go and to handle the trip without any medical problems.

My hair came back fuller than before, and in May I had my first haircut in eight months. Our summer in 2007 was probably the best we had since 2003. Pat and I enjoyed the pool and also entertaining on our new deck. We were particularly enjoying visits from our two grandchildren. My energy level was high and I was feeling better, both mentally and physically, than I had in years.

And I had three birthday parties! My birthday is the 4th of July, so there is always cause for celebration. But this year turned out to be special. I had a family party with my grandchildren and a neighborhood party where I annually get to cut the cake. Then, to top things off, I had a special surprise party from the Coldwell Banker office orchestrated by my wife, one of the agents and the office manager. It was totally unexpected. And everyone had a good time. I know that I did. I feel that my wife and I are truly blessed to have such a strong network of family and friends who are sincerely concerned about my wellbeing. *(See Lesson 7)*

We had a memorial service in Detroit in July for Pat's brother and came to some closure on his untimely death. On a happier note there, one of his daughters was expecting the first grandchild. And we were able to attend my sister, Janet, and her husband, Tom's 50th wedding anniversary in Indianapolis in August.

ANOTHER SETBACK/ FEELING LIKE JOB

However, my scans the end of August 2007 showed growth in the lung nodules for the first time since Nov 2006. Another setback.

I was quite discouraged since I had hoped that the chemo holiday would continue for some time to come. But that was not to be.

The largest nodule had grown back to the size it had when we started focusing on them in July 2006. It now looked like the chemo holiday had given the cancer a new chance to grow. Dr. Yi recommended that I immediately go back on chemo, and I started my treatments again the first week of September. When I started having the fatigue that comes with the chemo, I remembered how good I felt in the summer. And my hair started to fall out again, so, hopefully, that meant that the chemo was doing its job.

I was beginning to feel a bit like Job from the book in the Old Testament. We had studied it in my Thursday bible study group. If you are familiar with the story, Job was continually tested by Satan, and bad things kept happening to him. But his faith in the Lord helped him overcome adversity and he ended up stronger than before. If you are not familiar with the story, it is located a little over halfway through the Old Testament.

Dr. Yi told me that with nodules spread around my lungs, right side and left side, upper and lower, surgery was not a current option. He also advised that I needed to start thinking about my cancer as a chronic disease, like high blood pressure or diabetes: to be treated but not cured. Over time, we would use chemo as necessary in order to keep the nodules sub-centimeter in size and under control so they could not do much damage.

Also at this time, I started seeing Dr. Fong at Sloan Kettering twice a year for check-ups. Although I will bring him the latest results from the Princeton area machines, he always schedules CT scans at the Sloan Kettering facilities in NYC prior to the visit. I believe that he wants to get another view to confirm the scan findings. He advised me that surgery was not a current option, although he said that the robotic procedures are improving and at some time in the future, we might think about a surgical cure. But for the time being, he is very happy with my progress and as for the future, he said that, "We should let the tumors tell us what to do."

And, actually, my scans in November showed that the two largest nodules had indeed shrunk again to sub-centimeter size again so the plan was working. So for the time being, it looked like I would be on a program of six months on and then some time off. And, hopefully, this might work for a long time.

I recently talked to my wife about her feelings about this whole affair. She said that the one she had the most was the feeling of uncertainty. How long would I be around? Six months? Six years? Whatever? I agree that this is one of the most difficult feelings to manage with cancer and it is understandable. You don't really know if your next scan will show that the cancer has come back or maybe even spread.

But I told her that life itself is uncertain. And perhaps the cancer experience just brings that feeling to the forefront. We have both agreed that, while the feeling of uncertainty may not go away, what we can do is focus on living the best that we can today. We know that I am getting the best treatments that are available now and that the longer that I live, more treatments will be developed and approved. *(See Lesson 14)*

CHAPTER 15:
2008, The Chemo Merry-Go-Round

2008 was a year very similar to 2007. I was on chemo and the spots shrunk. Then I went on a holiday and after a while the spots grew again and I went back on chemo. With the fatigue and side effects of the chemo, life was basically a week on then a week off cycle. Since my second liver surgery, I had been on the same chemo merry-go-round for three years and it was getting a bit discouraging. I was beginning to realize that I may never be able to get off of the merry-go-round and would be on some sort of treatment for the rest of my life.

But the good news was that we were able to plan our life as we wanted to and not just around the chemo plan. We made a return trip to Paris in April and had a wonderful time. It was one of our best vacations. Then in June we were able to celebrate our 40th wedding anniversary with a party on our deck.

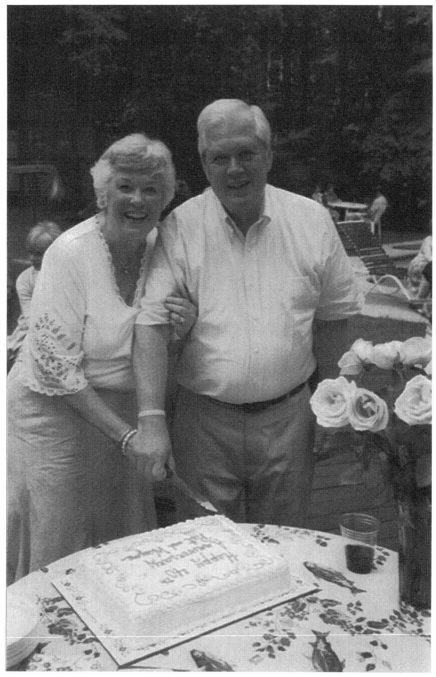

Cutting 40th Anniversary cake-June 2008

We also had a decent year in real estate and my wife made the NJAR Circle of Excellence again. And in November we spent Thanksgiving in Hong Kong with our daughter Kelly, who is now working there.

Perhaps the best thing for me for me was that I was able to continue singing in the Voices Chorale and the Methodist Church adult choir. As I have mentioned, I felt that singing was good for both my lungs and my mental attitude, and I felt that as long as I could sing pretty well, my lungs could not be in such bad shape.

———————

So I was beginning to feel pretty good about myself again. I was keeping the cancer under control and was enjoying life the best that I could. As I look at the cancer odds, the American Cancer Society stats for 2008 still continue to show a five-year success rate for stage IV colon cancer of about 10%. Not good. But odds are meant to be broken and someone has to do it. Based on how my treatment and results had progressed, there was no reason to believe that I should not be someone to beat the odds. I felt that over the previous five years, I had walked through the valley of the shadow of death, and I had come out safely on the other side. I had reached the far side of the survival curve. So why not me?

CHAPTER 16:
Planning for the Future

In 2009 I passed the five year threshold and had reached a new plateau in my treatments. There was no prescribed treatment for someone with stage IV colon cancer that had progressed so far, so with Dr. Yi's direction and Dr. Poplin's agreement, I started a maintenance treatment of Avastin-only every two weeks. So far I have not had the fatigue and side effects that came with the FOLFIRI regime. Our objective is to see if I do as well with Avastin-only as I did with the combined treatment. Maybe I can maintain a "new normal" with this treatment, which would be a good thing.

Pat and I recently attended a funeral in Charlotte, NC for one of my former IBM colleagues. While there I got into a discussion with one of the wives about my inclination to be always planning for the future. I thought about it a bit more and realized that it is an important part of dealing with cancer. If you are working on a non-cancer related future event, whether it is going out for dinner with friends, attending a concert or play, visiting the grandkids, going on a vacation trip and whether it is a day, a week, a month or even a year in advance, it takes your mind off of cancer. And the less time you spend thinking about your cancer, the more time you have to devote to more worthwhile pursuits. *(See Lesson 13)*

To illustrate that point, in May 2009, with the approval of Dr. Yi, Pat and I took our first Elderhostel trip to Florence, Italy where we spent nine days studying Renaissance Art and Architecture. A truly wonderful experience. And in June I spent a week with a group of 40 singers, mostly music professionals, in the Princeton Festival Choral Workshop where we rehearsed the Durufle Requiem and sang it in performance at the Princeton University Chapel. Another wonderful experience for me. And a good test of my voice.

My genes may also be helping me. While my father was slight of build and after a series of small strokes died peacefully in his sleep at the age of 76, my mother was a more Germanic build, was active teaching crafts at a nursing home well into her 80's and died at the age of 94. My build is more like my mothers, so maybe I inherited more of her genes and should be planning activities into my 90's.

I don't want to get arrogant about dealing with my cancer, since at any time, after any scan I may learn that it has come back stronger and in another place. But if that happens, hopefully, I will be able to deal with it with the treatments and procedures available at that time. In any case, as a precaution, in my financial planning analysis I have used my life expectancy to age 95.

CHAPTER 17:
Lessons Learned

So what have I learned? Here are some lessons that I picked up along the way that might be helpful to others. They are listed in the way that I thought about them and are not necessarily in a priority sequence.

LESSON 1: THE CAREGIVER

It is important to have a caregiver to support you during the process, and Pat has done an exceptional job in that capacity. She has gone with me for most of my consultations with Dr. Yi and all of my meetings with Dr. Fong and Dr. Poplin. Having two sets of ears hearing the advice makes it more likely that you will agree on the program going forward. She was also invaluable in helping me recover from the three surgeries, helping button and unbutton my shirts and letting me nap when I've been fatigued from chemotherapy.

LESSON 2: THE MEDICAL TEAM

I believe that I had the best medical care you could find. From Dr. Davidson's original colon surgery, to Dr. Poplin's advice, to Dr. Chandler's consultations, to Dr. Fong's liver surgeries, and most importantly to the knowledge, consultation, and humanity of Dr. Yi, I was blessed with the best advice that I could hope to find. I truly believe that without the knowledge and dedication of these people, I would not be here today.

LESSON 3: HAVING A PLAN

It's been said that when you don't know where you are going, any road will take you there. When you have a plan then you have some purpose in your life. We found that when we knew what was on the docket for the next month or two, it made living day by day much easier and just a step in the direction of the plan. And each good day that you have continues to build up your memories of the past. As they used to say at IBM, "Plan your work, and work your plan."

LESSON 4: KEEP THE FAITH, BABY

I have found that keeping the church involved in all the aspects of my journey has been very beneficial to me. From the church prayer chain that has prayed for the success of my surgeries and treatments, to the personal visitations from our senior pastor to the joy I have found in singing in the choir, to the Thursday small group meetings, to the daily prayers that my wife and I share, we have found strength in keeping our faith.

Our previous minister, Dr. Greg Young, frequently prayed with me for the healing touch of the Lord, and visited us both at home and in the hospitals in Princeton and NYC. This faith may have started in my early days in Bowling Green, Ohio, when my mother would dress up all of her children in their Sunday best and we would walk the four blocks to the local Methodist Church and take up a row of eight: mom and dad, and the six children. This was normally followed by a typical Sunday afternoon dinner, with, perhaps, one or two of my father's students in attendance.

A Bible verse which I have found particularly relevant to my current situation is found in Isaiah Chapter 40, verse 31. "But they that wait upon the Lord shall renew their strength; they shall mount up with wings as eagles; they shall run and not be weary; and they shall walk and not faint." Very well said.

LESSON 5: IT'S NOT YOUR FAULT

Cancer patients have a tendency to second guess the past. I know that I did. Why did this happen to me? What did I do wrong? But that kind of thinking does not help in your treatment or in the outcome. Getting cancer is not your fault. You just have to know that those kinds of things happen in life, and your objective now is not to dwell on what might have been but on what is. So I believe the best option is to get your plan in place and stick with it. Don't think about who is to blame. Think about your actions.

LESSON 6: YOU'VE GOT TO HAVE HOPE

There is a song in the musical Damn Yankees called "You've got to have heart" sung by the Washington baseball team in the locker room regarding their game with the Yankees. One line in the song goes. "You've got to have hope; mustn't sit around and mope." And that is true with the fight against cancer. You have got to hope that you will succeed. You have got to hope that tomorrow will be better than today. You have got to have hope that the treatment will work. If you don't have hope in what you are doing, than the odds are that it will be a self-fulfilling prophecy and you will fail.

I am now wearing a yellow Livestrong Bracelet from the Lance Armstrong Foundation. Any time during the day that I feel that I am losing my confidence or feeling down about things, I take a look at the bracelet and it reminds me that I must have hope.

LESSON 7: DON'T HIDE IT

I found that talking about my situation was better than hiding it. As I mentioned earlier, we had a pretty good sized email base that we updated after major events in my journey. I keep the Thursday group up to date on my progress. All of our local friends knew about my condition. We talked openly to other church members in the church coffee hour, a number of whom have had their own cancer experiences.

One day I counted five church members coming in or going out of my oncologist's offices.

The one area of our lives that we did not talk about it much was to our real estate customers. As long as we were able to provide good service, we did not want to jeopardize relationships or business dealings by having customers worrying about my condition. Some of our customers knew about my condition, but many of them did not. Those that did were supportive of us and always interested in my wellbeing.

LESSON 8: THE MIND VS. THE BODY

My Brother Jim's philosophy regarding controlling the mental part of your life has stuck with me throughout my treatment. You can't worry about the how's and why's of cancer, which is the physical side of things. What you can control is your response which is the mental side of things. His motto is,"I don't have Parkinson's. My body does." The same statement could be just as true with cancer.

LESSON 9: KEEP A POSITIVE MENTAL ATTITUDE

Somewhere along my IBM career, I went to a seminar entitled "Success Through A Positive Mental Attitude." It focused our own ability to determine what our mental attitude is going to be at any point in time and on our need to have a positive attitude every day. I have mentioned earlier that people have commented to me about my positive attitude. I believe that, whether you are dealing with cancer or something else in your life, a daily positive attitude is one of the most important things that you can bring to the table.

LESSON 10: KNOW YOUR STUFF

I have found that the more you know about your specific cancer and your treatments the better off you are, the better questions you can ask your oncologist and surgeon, and the more likely you are to understand their responses. As I mentioned earlier, I searched out a lot of information on the internet regarding colon cancer and its treatments. I am even signed up for a service that distributes results of presentations from some of the annual meetings of the oncologists. And I download the annual reports of the American Cancer Society. I have subscribed to Cure, a magazine dedicated to cancer education, and I pick up the pharma brochures on the various chemos that I take. I also get a lot of side information from the chemo nurses. It makes me feel good to know that I have a little bit of the knowledge it takes to understand the cancer that I have.

LESSON 11: TAKE CONTROL

When you have knowledge about your cancer and its treatments, you have a chance to take control of your situation. Not that you are going to be your own oncologist or surgeon, but that you are going to know what treatments you are on, what your treatment options are, what your treatment schedule is going to be, when your next scans are going to be scheduled and any other activities that might be necessary for your treatment. This is all part of the strategy to learn to control your cancer and not let your cancer control you.

LESSON 12: EXPECT THE UNEXPECTED

Things won't go as you have planned. Just when you think that things will be getting back to a more normal situation, you will probably get some unexpected news. The cancer will have outwitted you again. So you need to expect surprises. That is why it is very important to have your plan in place and stick with it. There may be bumps along the road, but you can learn to deal with them. Expect the abnormal to be the normal and you won't get as discouraged when it happens.

LESSON 13: PLANNING FOR THE FUTURE

Planning non-cancer related events for some time in the future helps to take your mind off of the problems with your current condition. And that is a positive thing. If you are actively thinking about an event next week, next month or even next year, you have less time to think about your disease. It almost doesn't matter what it is; a dinner out, a trip to NYC for a play, or a vacation trip to Europe. Having the events on the calendar will get you to thinking about them and may even increase your motivation to "make it to the date." And once reaching the event successfully, you can then make more plans for the future. The more time that you spend on planning non-cancer related events and the less time you spend thinking about your disease, the better off you will be.

LESSON 14: A DAY AT A TIME

It may sound a little cliché to say it, but you have to take the journey a day at a time. Getting stage IV colon cancer, or any serious cancer or disease for that matter, is not a good thing. But with the treatments available today you can, hopefully, hang on for a long time. That's what I hope happens to me. So what you have to do is take the day you have today and make the best of it. You can't do anything more about yesterday and you can have a plan for tomorrow, but today is the day that you can actually make something happen.

CHAPTER 18:
Bonus Time, On the Far Side of the Curve

So there you have it. My journey started in 2003 but is, I hope, far from over in 2009. I am still standing after almost six years. As I previously mentioned, recently several oncologists have told me that I am "on the far side of the curve," that I am "one of a kind," and that I am "unique." Several doctors have personally admitted to me that they just did not expect me to be around this long. When your doctors start talking to you openly in those terms, maybe there is some truth to it. Maybe I am indeed a "Miracle Man." And since there is no established chemo protocol for someone who has survived so long, my treatment is "unique" as well and may establish some guidance for those who come along after me.

So as I see it, if my doctors did not expect me to live this long, then every day for me is a bonus and I am essentially on "Bonus Time." This is not "Borrowed Time," that would have to be paid back, but "Bonus Time" which is extra time that you were not expected to have in your life. And that is pretty exciting.

I don't recall any single "aha" moment or tipping point when I realized that I was indeed on the far side of the survival curve. Looking back it is also hard for me to believe that I really have gone through all that I have in the past six years. But I realize that it is a culmination of a lot of things that were just taken one step at a time and one day at a time.

And it is also somewhat paradoxical and ironic to analyze what I have been through when you consider that I started with Stage IV cancer just three years after a normal colonoscopy. That would have to put me on or close to the near side of the curve when I was first diagnosed. So I have experienced both sides of the curve. Just amazing, when you think about it.

I am beginning to realize that in the grand scheme of cancer patients I am indeed unique in my experience and probably really have achieved something special. Every time I read in the newspaper about some notable individual who has died from cancer after maybe a year or two of treatments, I realize how blessed I am. I also believe that I have an obligation to use my experience for the benefit of others. To give them hope as well.

So I try to live every day to the fullest. Because of the neuropathy in my feet and hands, I am limited in some of the things that I used to enjoy doing such as mixed doubles tennis, playing folk songs on the guitar at parties, and going for long walks with our collie, Luke. There are, however, other things that I can enjoy in their place. These include swimming, singing, attending concerts, reading American history books, traveling, doing Sudoku math puzzles, and, would you believe it, even bird watching and stamp collecting. And Pat and I really enjoy grandparenting with Xavier and Rafael.

I would have to say that I am very proud of Xavier in his courageous and, so far, successful fight against leukemia. I went up to help out with his chemo a couple of times at the Morristown Memorial Hospital where his watchword was "No ouchies." He has also become the "poster child" for several organizations and fund raisers, most recently the Valerie Fund, and made his debut on national television in support of a fund walk.

If everything goes well, next spring he will complete his three year treatment program.

I have also thought about taking up bridge again. In college I played bridge for spending money and was pretty good at the play of the cards. Pat & I played a lot in Holland and Hong Kong, but it kind of gave way to other things over time. So maybe with a refresher course on bidding, I could take it up again. Scott and I have frequently engaged again in the father-son chess matches that we used to enjoy years ago. Also I have told Pat that I would continue to support her in real estate as long as she cares to work.

So I have more than enough things to do to keep my mind off of cancer. And I do find that this year I am thinking a lot less about my cancer than I did several years ago. It is mostly when I am entering the medical building once every two weeks for an infusional treatment that I realize again that I am indeed a cancer patient, and a survivor. Other than that, I don't think much about it at all. Life is pretty stable. Obviously, that could change with my next scans but that is how I feel now.

I have enjoyed writing this because it has helped me remember all of the support that I have had in living through this experience. It has helped me remember many of the good things in my life and has helped strengthen my resolve in dealing with this life changing and threatening disease. It has also helped me to realize how fortunate I have been to have come this far, to have reached the far side of the curve as a cancer survivor, and has encouraged me to continue to go forward with renewed hope, strength, and purpose for the future.

If you or someone you know is just starting on a cancer journey or perhaps has another difficult disease, I trust that this story will give you some hope that things can also go well for you along the path. So far, the path has gone well for me. With the support of my wife, my children, family, friends and doctors, I feel truly blessed and, God willing, I will keep on going, planning for the future and enjoying life and my Bonus Time; " On the Far Side of the Curve."

Author's Notes

I wrote this story myself over a period of about two years from the summer of 2007 to the summer of 2009 with occasional periods of intense thought followed by lapses when I had set the project aside. Crossing the five year mark helped energize me again.

While I may be responsible for the words, there are a number of people that I would like to thank for helping me out with my thought process, organization, editing, sentence structure, chapter headings and any number of things which, I hope, have helped make this a better book than it would be if I had done it alone. These include my wife Pat, my children Scott and Kelly, Scott's wife Cristina, my brother Jim, Dr. Yi, and a number of doctors, friends and church members, specifically Jack Taylor, Barbara Fox, and Tim and Linda Henry, all of whom helped me along the way.

I would also like to give my thanks to Richard K. Rein, editor and publisher of U.S. 1 Newspaper, Princeton's business and entertainment weekly, who saw the value of my story and gave me unexpected encouragement when he published an early version of it in the newspaper on December 19, 2007.

At that time he wrote, "The author of our first person feature, Wayne Cooke, at first might seem more like a person who would need help rather than give it. Yet his exposition of his four-year battle with cancer is both heartening and helpful."

And finally I would like to give thanks to photographer Craig Terry, who illustrated that publication and provided the cover photograph for this book.

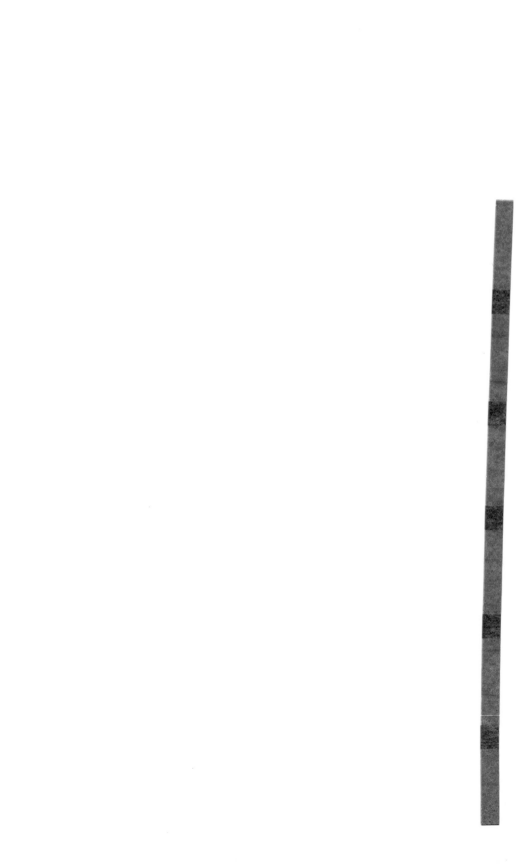

Marshall Co Public Library
ie Benton
1003 Poplar Street
Benton, KY 42025

**Marshall Co Public Library
@ Benton
1003 Poplar Street
Benton, KY 42025**

5937941R0

Made in the USA
Charleston, SC
23 August 2010